Group and

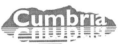

of related interest

The Activity Year Book
A Week by Week Guide for Use in Elderly Day and Residential Care
Annie Bowden and Nancy Lewthwaite
ISBN 978 1 84310 963 1

The Pool Activity Level (PAL) Instrument for Occupational Profiling
A Practical Resource for Carers of People with Cognitive Impairment
3rd edition
Jackie Pool
ISBN 978 1 84310 594 7

Group and Individual Work with Older People

A Practical Guide to Running Successful Activity-based Programmes

Swee Hong Chia, Julie Heathcote and
Jane Marie Hibberd

Illustrated by Andrew J. Hibberd

Jessica Kingsley *Publishers*
London and Philadelphia

First published 2011
by Jessica Kingsley Publishers
116 Pentonville Road
London N1 9JB, UK
and
400 Market Street, Suite 400
Philadelphia, PA 19106, USA

www.jkp.com

Library of Congress Cataloging in Publication Data
Chia, Swee Hong.
Group and individual work with older people : a practical guide to running successful activity-based programmes / Swee Hong Chia, Julie Healthcote and Jane Marie Hibberd ; illustrated by Andrew J. Hibberd.
p. cm.
Includes bibliographical references and index.
ISBN 978-1-84905-128-6 (alk. paper)
1. Older people--Services for. 2. Older people--Health and hygiene. 3. Older people--Mental health. 4. Social work with older people. I. Healthcote, Julie. II. Hibberd, Jane Marie. III. Title.
HV1451.C44 2012
362.6068--dc23
2011020218

British Library Cataloguing in Publication Data
A CIP catalogue record for this book is available from the British Library

ISBN 978 1 84905 128 6

Printed and bound in Great Britain

Contents

List of Figures

List of Tables

Disciaimers

Although every effort has been made, it is not possible to trace or contact all sources of material reproduced in this book, and we therefore regret any inadvertent omission of acknowledgement where it is due.

All names and place references used within this book are fictional and any reference to known names of persons or place names is entirely coincidental.

Acknowledgements

We would like to thank older people, colleagues and students who have inspired us and our families who have supported us. We would also like to thank the following for their advice and help with materials for this book: Elizabeth Patricia Walker, Maggie Woodhouse, Alison Begley, Moira Clare, Elizabeth Henderson, Garry Nightingale and Ryan Jones.

Introduction

Activity is fundamental to all human well-being and existence, including in older age. On a daily basis, people will engage in many activities such as dressing, preparing food, eating, going out, communicating, relaxing, caring for others and going to sleep. Although these activities may not necessarily be done in the same manner or with the same level of enthusiasm, engagement in activity gives meaning to people's lives. Some activities can be done alone, as reading the newspaper, or they can be completed in pairs or in groups, such as chatting with friends, visiting the shops or a local club. The urge to participate in activities can be considered a basic human need. This inner motivation does not diminish as an individual grows older, but the common effects of ageing, such as reduced vision, increased incidence of medical conditions – for example, arthritis or dementia – and social aspects such as loneliness can affect an individual's level of engagement with activities. Some of the effects of ageing can be minimised by a warm and supportive environment, caring staff, careful assessment and provision of appropriate activities and, if appropriate, equipment (College of Occupational Therapists and National Association for Providers of Activities for Older People 2007).

The purpose of this book is to help facilitators or staff who are working with older people and:

- want to know more about the value of activities
- are aware of the importance of activities but do not know how to initiate group or individual work
- want to run groups efficiently and successfully
- are keen to set up activity-based groups but find they encounter challenges in the running of such groups
- want to maintain creativity in groups

- are keen to evaluate and improve their work.

There are three types of groups: activity groups emphasise the task or end product of the group, support groups value sharing and group process dimensions, and psychotherapy groups aim to help members gain insight and explore their feelings (Finlay 2000). This book will focus on the development of the first two groups – first, activity groups: for example, reminiscence groups and arts and crafts groups, which aim to maintain or develop individuals' skills such as hand-eye co-ordination; and, second, support and communication groups: for example, discussion and life skills groups, which encourage group members to give each other support and share experiences. Both aims may exist in any one group – for example, a member who is baking a cake may also be using the time to reminisce about their first experience of cooking. By focusing on activity and support groups, this book will address the issues that need to be considered when initiating, establishing, running and evaluating individual and group work with older people within their homes, supported living, community centres, dementia cafés and hospitals.

While each chapter provides theoretical knowledge and examples, there is a greater focus on the practical elements that include the following.

- A single case study, Betty, which is used throughout the book to link the key themes and provide an example to help facilitators consider and address appropriate practices that meet individual needs.

- A variety of case studies, which provide illustrations of older people's responses and examples of good practice in group and individual work.

- A series of exercises, which can be used for reflective practice. These could be used for training purposes and staff development.

CHAPTER 1

Quality of Life in Older Age

What is quality of life?

According to the University of Toronto (2010), quality of life is 'the degree to which a person enjoys the important possibilities of his or her life'. Enjoyment consists of two components: the experience of satisfaction or the achievement of some characteristics as indicated by the expression 'she enjoys good health'.

The University of Toronto have suggested the following framework, which comprises three life domains, each of which is subdivided into three subdomains:

1. **Being: who one is**

    (a) Physical being – for example, physically able to get around one's home and neighbourhood.

    (b) Psychological being – for example, coping with what life brings.

    (c) Spiritual being – for example, feeling that one's life is accomplishing something.

2. **Belonging: connections with one's environment**

    (a) Physical belonging – for example, living in a place especially equipped for seniors.

    (b) Social belonging – for example, having neighbours one can turn to.

    (c) Community belonging – for example, going to places in one's neighbourhood.

3. Becoming: achievable personal goals, hopes and aspirations

(a) Practical becoming – for example, doing work around one's home such as cleaning and cooking.

(b) Leisure becoming – for example, participating in organised leisure activities.

(c) Growth becoming – for example, adjusting to changes in one's personal life.

The extent of an individual's quality of life in the domains of being, belonging and becoming is determined by two factors: importance and enjoyment. Quality of life equates the relative importance or meaning attached to each particular domain and the extent of the individual's enjoyment with respect to each domain. In this way, the quality of life is adapted to the life of every individual at any time and from their individual perspective, and can be affected by such factors as a person's social class, ethnicity, gender and geographical locations in certain cases. However, researchers at the University of Toronto are concerned that some individuals – for example, older people living in institutions – may perceive their quality of life to be satisfactory because they have had little opportunity to experience other possibilities or empowerment to make any changes (Quality of Life Research Unit 2010). To address this potential problem, these researchers have proposed that a quality environment provides basic needs – that is, food, shelter, safety and social contact, opportunities within the individual's potential and control, and choice within the environment.

Mountain (2004) suggested that the contributory factors to the quality of life in older age include sufficient income, maintenance of health, involvement in meaningful activities and extent of social contact. Impaired social engagement has been linked with a variety of health problems. Spending time alone, being widowed, single or divorced and having impaired mental health are among the vulnerability factors for loneliness (Victor *et al.* 2004). Owen (2006) reinforced the need for meaningful activities that can provide a sense of purpose and a continued role in life.

The National Institute for Health and Clinical Excellence (NICE) (2008) suggested that the key factors affecting the mental health and well-being of older people are discrimination, participation in meaningful activities, relationships, physical health and poverty. Allen (2008) found evidence that many older people are becoming more dissatisfied, feeling lonelier and more depressed, which could subsequently impact on their satisfaction with life and well-being.

Bowling *et al.* (2003) suggested the following: individuals should be encouraged to develop positive thinking and direct their perception upwards, to learn to be and to feel more in control of their everyday lives and competing demands. These will enhance the coping skills of individuals as they grow older.

How does the ageing process affect quality of life?

The ageing process (normal ageing) represents the universal biological changes that occur with age and are unaffected by disease and environmental influences. Not all of these age-related changes have an adverse impact on day-to-day activity. The process of ageing is strongly influenced by the effects of environmental, lifestyle and disease states that in turn are related to or change with ageing but are not the result of ageing itself. Byers-Connon, Lohman and Padilla (2004) pointed out that a definition of health is the absence of disease or other abnormal condition. Very few older people would be considered healthy with this definition. They said:

> However, a theory of well-being can be developed if health is considered the optimal level of functioning for a person's age and condition. Many individuals have chronic illnesses to which they have adjusted and are able to live optimally. These people could be considered to be in a state of well-being.

The Alzheimer's Society (2010) stressed that quality of life is possible following a dementia diagnosis. The 'My Name is not Dementia' report found that, in the sample concerned, people rated relationships or someone to talk to and the ability to communicate as key indicators of their quality of life. The report concluded that many factors (outside dementia) affect a person's quality of life and such an approach could be applicable to older people with other health or social needs.

The International Classification of Functioning, Disability and Health

The International Classification of Functioning, Disability and Health, known more commonly as the 'ICF', is a classification of health and health-related domains. These domains are classified from body, individual and societal perspectives by means of a series of lists: body functions and structure, and a list of domains of activity and participation. Because an individual's functioning and disability occurs within a specific situation, the ICF also includes a list of environmental factors. The ICF is the World Health Organization's (WHO) framework for measuring health and disability at both individual and population levels.

The ICF captures the notions of 'health' and 'disability' in a new light. It acknowledges that every human being can experience a decline in health and some degree of disability. The ICF takes into account the social aspects of disability and does not see disability only as a 'medical' or 'biological' dysfunction. By including contextual factors, in which environmental factors are listed, the ICF allows one to record the impact of the environment on a person's functioning. An extensive examination of the ICF can be found in Davis (2006). Please see below for an example of identifying the impact of a health condition to some of the ICF concepts:

> **Health condition, disorder or disease:** dementia – Alzheimer's disease
>
> **Body function, structure and impairment:** brain – memory
>
> **Activity limitation:** unable to remember things
>
> **Participation restriction:** gradual loss of roles with daily living skills

> **Health condition, disorder or disease:** arthritis: rheumatoid arthritis
>
> **Body function, structure and impairment:** hands – pain and development of contractures
>
> **Activity limitation:** unable to hold things
>
> **Participation restriction:** gradual loss of ability to hold utensils

Person-centred care and quality of life

In recent years there has been considerable interest in person-centred care, which aims to maintain the personhood of individuals and in particular those with dementia (Kitwood 1997). Kitwood considers personhood as 'a standing or a status that is bestowed on one human being by another in the context of relationship and social being' (Kitwood 1997, p.8). Stokes and Goudie (2003) noted that, within person-centred care, carers and facilitators should accept older people with dementia as unique individuals who have a life history, and that they should acknowledge each person's experience of the condition. Woodhouse (2006) noted that a barrier to the achievement of person-centred care is the unrelenting double stigma that surrounds older people with dementia. This stigma has arisen because of society's attitude towards ageing and the social construction of dementia. Based on her experience, Woodhouse suggested that one of the most successful strategies for challenging stereotypical attitudes is to invite individuals with dementia to participate in staff training.

Although person-centred care is particularly significant for individuals with dementia, the principles are useful and relevant for all older people. The Dignity in Care Campaign (Department of Health 2006) stresses the importance of treating people as individuals and points out that the dignity of older people includes respecting their privacy, autonomy and self-worth. Dignity Champions aim to improve care standards (Department of Health 2006). A person-centred approach aims to see individuals as people, rather than focusing on their illness or abilities they may have lost. Instead of treating the individual as a collection of symptoms and behaviours to be managed, person-centred care considers the whole person, taking into account each individual's unique qualities, abilities, interests, preferences and needs. Person-centred care also means treating individuals with dignity and respect, which includes:

- seeking to understand the individual
- helping the person feel valued
- respecting cultural values
- acting with courtesy
- respecting privacy

- helping people feel good about themselves

- offering simple choices.

The approach stresses that respect is maintained by:

- creating situations in which older people, as individuals, are likely to succeed; selecting activities that they can still manage and enjoy; offering encouragement and support; and letting them do things at their own pace, if appropriate (of particular importance is the engagement with activities that help people retain their independence)

- breaking activities down into small steps so that people gain a sense of achievement, even if they can only manage part of a task

- encouraging people to take pride in their appearance, and complimenting them on doing this (Alzheimer's Society 2010a).

Exercise: Assessing a day in terms of quality of life

Consider a typical day and use the activity chart to indicate the main activity you are likely to be doing within each half-hour. It is unlikely that you will be able to complete this within a continuous 24-hour period.

Activity chart

Time	Activity	On own	With others (If so, with whom?)
6.00 a.m.	Waking up, washing and dressing	Yes	
6.30 a.m.	Preparing breakfast	Yes	
7.00 a.m.	Waiting for the bus	No	Yes – with another working colleague
7.30 a.m.	Travelling and talking	No	As above
8.00 a.m.	Travelling and talking	No	As above
8.30 a.m.	Having a cup of coffee	No	As above
9.00 a.m.	Bathing client	Yes	
9.30 a.m.	Bathing client	Yes	
10.00 a.m.	Bathing client	Yes	
10.30 a.m.	Bathing client	Yes	
11.00 a.m.	Laying table	No	Yes – with another working colleague
11.30 a.m.	Helping client with eating	No	Yes – with other clients and staff
12.00 noon	Helping client with eating	No	Yes – with other clients and staff
12.30 p.m.	Helping client with eating	No	Yes – with other clients and staff
1.00 p.m.	Having lunch and socialising	No	Yes – with two other staff
1.30 p.m.			
2.00 p.m.			
2.30 p.m.			
3.00 p.m.			
3.30 p.m.			
4.00 p.m.			
4.30 p.m.			
5.00 p.m.			
5.30 p.m.			

Calculate the number of hours you spend on your own and with others. Are you happy with the results? Is it an accurate reflection of your daily schedule? You could then complete this exercise again for an older person.

Using analysis to consider quality of life

A Strengths Weaknesses Opportunities Barriers (SWOB) analysis is a useful tool for identifying positive and negative issues against the backdrop of external opportunities and barriers or threats (Atkinson 2004). It could be used to analyse an older person's individual day in a care home or the staff's practice, or a facilitator could use it for a group in the community. It offers a snapshot of practice. Choose one of the following analyses: physical environment, individual's day, staff – individual interaction, and individual–individual interaction. This is a useful exercise for team work to assess quality of life factors.

A completed example of a SWOB analysis of a physical environment in a care home is as follows.

Strengths
Pleasant communal living room

Weaknesses
Worn-out furniture
Walls need a fresh coat of paint

Opportunities
Enthusiastic staff
Willing volunteers

Barriers
Shortage of staff

Use the following goal-setting format to achieve your plan:
Goal: to decorate the living room before the end of the year.
Strategies and resources: ask individuals; seek the help of volunteers; consider fund raising; approach local DIY companies for donation of decorating materials.
Evidence: living room decorated by the end of the year.
Achieved and dated: if not, why not? How could this be resolved?

The following case study of Betty will be used in most of the chapters to help link some of the key themes and provide examples to help facilitators consider and address appropriate practice that meets the group and individual needs of older people.

Case study: Betty

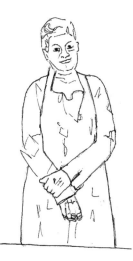

Betty is an 80-year-old English woman. She comes from a small, supportive family. Her early days were spent in China. She returned to England when she was 12 years old. She enjoyed rowing. She did well at school and achieved a teaching diploma. She was married for 40 years and has one son, Sam. She worked as a teacher in her local primary school until her retirement. She receives a pension and lives in a semi-detached house. She needs glasses for reading small print. She wears a hearing aid. She is fit and takes regular exercise. She is outgoing and relates to people well. Until recently, Betty's life has revolved around her local community through the Women's Institute.

Over the last few years, Betty has become easily confused and developed short-term memory loss, which is getting progressively worse. She has given up housework. Before admission, there were a couple of times when a saucepan caught fire because Betty forgot to turn off an electric ring. Sam had to check that Betty was appropriately dressed. She might occasionally use the large plant pot as a toilet. Betty's friends found it difficult to understand her. Sam was also finding it stressful to cope with the needs of his mother at home. He wondered if his mother was depressed.

Betty has since been admitted to a local care home. She has also been diagnosed with Alzheimer's disease and prescribed with Aricept.

Exercise

Using the case study of Betty, consider the following questions regarding her quality of life:

Which aspects of the changes in Betty are attributable to the ageing process?

Which aspects of Betty's behaviour could be due to Alzheimer's disease?

What actions could be undertaken to improve Betty's quality of life?

What could be done to maintain Betty's quality of life?

CHAPTER 2

Group and Individual Work

What are the functions of group and individual work?

Group work

According to Bender, Norris and Bauckham (1994), a group consists of individuals of all ages who are classed together because they have some purpose or needs. Garvin, Gutierrez and Galinsky (2004) have suggested that group work can enhance function, ameliorate problems, produce social change and promote social justice. Walsh (1993) believed that participation in regular groups fosters a sense of belonging and togetherness. Leary (1994) noted that individuals may find companionship, feel supported and gain a sense of belonging through sharing their concerns and difficulties. This may be of a particular significance to older people.

Group work is not totally unproblematic, however. One challenge is that individuals may receive less attention and their privacy may be compromised. The Department of Health (2003) pointed out that, while some individuals want an active, well-organised social life, others prefer a level of privacy and want independence from others. Finlay (2000) also pointed out that group experiences are powerful and can therefore be beneficial as well as destructive. As a result, facilitators need to be able to manage with sensitivity the complex dynamics generated where interdependent people relate to one another – for example, older people living in care homes. However, Bender *et al.* (1994) added that groups do not solve all problems presented by older people.

In a longitudinal study of 2761 men and women in America, Glass *et al.* (1999) suggested a link between 'social and productive occupation such as attending church and going out to restaurants' and survival. Analysis showed that those older people who were less active were more likely to die earlier than those who were more active. Mountain and Moore (1995) found that the activities and social atmosphere of a day centre helped less active individuals and reduced their feelings of loneliness.

Tester *et al.* (2004) undertook a quality of life study with 52 residents with severe physical or mental health conditions. The residents expressed the following concerns: inability to feel at home and to express their sense of self and their need for privacy; need for some control over daily living; requirement to fit in with rules and timetables and being unsupported in a basic activity; and need for social interaction for sense of self, development and maintenance of relationships with other residents, and quality of life. Factors that can maintain self-esteem include strong family support, inner resources, long-established ability to cope and receiving appropriate interventions. While engagement with stimulating and purposeful activities gives individuals some sense of self, being able to opt out from organised activities should always be possible.

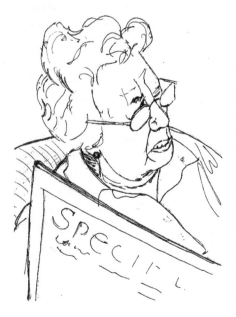

Group work can help to alleviate the isolation and loneliness that can exist in hospitals and individual care homes. A systematic review by Cattan *et al.* (2005) defines loneliness as an expression of an individual's sense of aloneness. Social isolation was seen to involve the lack of social contact. The review illustrated that group-based activities helped to alleviate both loneliness and social isolation. Of the ten interventions that were effective, none of them were group-based. The review stressed that a common factor for all successful group-based activities is that older people contribute in some way to the planning and development of the activities.

Individual work

As the book is also about individual work, it is essential to consider the needs of older people who do not enjoy being part of a group – for example, they may be threatened by the size of the group or the level of noise created. Being with other individuals does not necessarily reduce feelings such as depression especially if the individuals feel that they do not fit in with the aims and the needs of other people in the group. It is important to ensure that what individuals wish to do is considered in any session whether it is group or individual based.

The feelings of helplessness associated with long-term disability can affect motivation levels, which are hampered if there is a lack of structure and meaning to an individual's day. These feelings can be minimised by a motivating and supportive environment with opportunities for interaction and engagement in meaningful activities on a one-to-one basis or during group work. Individual work for a short period of time may be more appropriate and beneficial for individuals who are frail (Owen 2006). Brooker (2001) indicated that some individuals need to feel useful and engaged in meaningful activities by, for example, participating in household activities instead of timetabled activities in care homes. Perrin, May and Anderson (2010) emphasised the importance of being aware of the quieter, less demanding individuals who may be starved of human contact. Their well-being may be enhanced by contact that is both frequent and brief.

Walsh (1993) commented that some individuals may need peace and quiet and may not function in a group setting that could be viewed as confusing and noisy. Some groups are not always suitable if individuals have difficulty contributing and have poor group work skills (Leary 1994). Mountain (2004) observed that there is an expectation for individuals to interact and participate in group activities. Yet this may not be what the individual wants, one reluctant day hospital group service user describing it as 'They will be having groups and being noisy'. Heathcote (2005) pointed out that some individuals may not be suited to some types of groups because of poor hearing, confusion or frailty. For them, such an approach can be threatening and they may prefer to work in their own space, in a more private way.

It is therefore important to view people as individuals and to use knowledge from informal and formal assessments to consider if the individual needs are best met through individual or group work, or ideally a combination of both. While some groups do offer support to each individual, it is also important that participants are allowed ownership of their group and the development of ideas and activities. This should be the case with groups in both the community and care settings. The Commission for Social Care Inspection (CSCI 2006) stated that the care of older people in care homes should be individualised and not institutionalised. The Care Quality Commission (2009) emphasised the need for individuals to be involved in planning their care, with information provided to enable them to make informed choices and their being supported to live as independently as possible.

BENEFITS OF INDIVIDUAL WORK

Most group activities can be adapted to a one-to-one setting. Individual work – for example, reminiscence – can take many forms such as working on a life story book, making a memory board, one-to-one talking and recording of memories, or the recall of memories without an end product. One of the major advantages of individual work is the undivided attention that can be given to each individual, thus allowing the person to attend and to concentrate on the activity with minimum distraction, as in learning to use a computer. Facilitators will gain a better understanding of the strengths and needs of the individual by questioning and offering appropriate support. Individual work complements group work because it can assist the individual in promoting independence, self-maintenance, dignity and choice, which in turn enhances well-being. Where appropriate, it is important to encourage individuals in care settings to continue with their hobbies and interests so that life can remain as normal and enjoyable as possible, despite their change in circumstances. Cultural sensitivity is also an important component in planning activities (Mold, Fitzpatrick and Roberts 2005). MacBrayne (2007) suggested that offering individuals the opportunity to engage in familiar activities such as food preparation could be motivating and give them the added benefit of a desirable end product. Owen (2006) recommended engagement with the outside world, because it is essential to ensure that residents in care settings still feel part of the community.

Case study: Marion

A recent illness left Marion weak and unable to leave her room in the nursing home. Pauline, one of the nurses, was concerned that she was isolated, spending long periods on her own and missing the group activities in the lounge. Following a poetry-reading session, Pauline decided to take the poetry book to Marion's room to see if she would like to hear some of the poems. Marion chose several poems that she remembered learning at school and Pauline read them to her. Marion was able to join in with the words; she smiled and enjoyed talking to Pauline about her childhood. For a little while Marion forgot her illness and Pauline found out information about her that she had not known before.

Case study: Betty

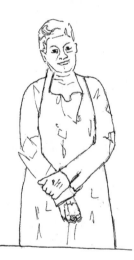

Suzie, one of the nurses, was concerned that Betty seemed isolated and missed the group activities in the lounge. Suzie learned from the notes that Betty had worked as a primary school teacher. She asked Betty if she would like to read short stories for the local school. Although initially reluctant, Betty was willing to try. She was particularly pleased when she read a story without any prompting.

EXAMPLES OF INDIVIDUAL WORK

An individual programme of work can range from an informal to a formalised method of writing down the details of the work involved. The latter is based on the behavioural approach. This offers a structured method of writing programmes, which, once mastered, can be adapted to meet both informal and formal training programmes. This method of writing programmes is now described together with information about how the process can be adapted to produce a less formal programme. Individual work programmes must be based on an older person's assessed needs and interests. One of the major strengths of a formalised individual work programme with clearly defined objectives and methods is in maintaining continuity through staff changes. Individual and group work cannot take place in a vacuum but must be undertaken within a caring and nurturing work environment (Peck and Hong 1994).

This is a completed example.

Name: Amy

Activity: Making sandwich

Long-term goal: Amy will be able to make a jam sandwich

Current goal: Amy will spread jam on two slices of bread

Criterion for success: Amy will use a sufficient amount of jam for the two slices of bread

Procedure: You will need two slices of bread, butter, jam, a knife and a plate

Do this activity before coffee at 10.00 a.m.

Activities: Make sure Amy is seated upright with head in midline, hands on her lap or table, hips flexed and feet rested on foot rest.

To begin with, talk with Amy about the morning's activity. Place the ingredients in front of her. Begin the process by spreading butter on the bread. Ask her to spread jam on the two slices of bread. Praise her if she picks up the knife, uses a sufficient amount of jam and spreads it on the two slices of bread.

If she does not respond, remind her of the activity and hold her wrist to complete the task i.e. spreading jam on the two slices of bread. Praise her. Ask her if she would like to eat her sandwich.

Date:

Comments: Amy was enthusiastic but needed a lot of support to complete the task. She appeared tired.

Initials:

Here is another completed example of an individual work programme using a different format.

Name: Sunny

Address:

Professionals involved: Occupational therapist

Date:

The points included below are not intended to be a full list of an individual's abilities and needs but are those areas that seem most helpful in guiding aims within the group. These aims will be reviewed regularly and revised when necessary.

Strengths: Sunny has some head control when he is seated.

Sunny can distinguish his carers and shows affection towards them. He can establish eye contact. He is generally alert and is aware of the left side of his body. He can let us know when he does not want to do something.

Needs: Sunny needs to develop awareness of the right side of his body.

The activities listed here should aim to meet the current needs of the individual identified in the strengths and needs list. First, specify the aim as briefly as possible and then describe activities that will help achieve this. Any special equipment or materials should also be mentioned so we can be appropriately prepared for each session.

Aim: to develop awareness of the right side of his body.

Activities: sit opposite Sunny. Place his arms on the table in front of him. Select and place one piece of reminiscence equipment in front of him. Aim to establish awareness of his right side by moving the equipment towards his right side.

Special materials: a special chair and a box of reminiscence based activities.

Comments: note the length of time Sunny pays attention when the equipment is moved towards the right side of his body.

This is an example of a work programme involving Betty.

Name: Betty

Address:

Professionals involved: Occupational therapist

Date:

The points included below are not intended to be a full list of an individual's abilities and needs but are those areas that seem most helpful in guiding therapy aims within the group. These aims will be reviewed regularly and revised when necessary.

Strengths: Betty can distinguish her carers and shows affection towards them. She can establish eye contact. She is generally alert and is fairly communicative particularly in the mornings.

Needs: Betty needs to continue to orientate in time by means of daily newspapers.

The activities listed here should aim to meet the current needs of the individual identified in the strengths and needs list. First, specify the aim as briefly as possible and then describe activities that will help achieve this. Any special equipment or materials should also be mentioned so we can be appropriately prepared for each session.

Aim: to maintain time orientation by means of newspapers.

Activities: sit beside Betty. Place the newspapers in front of her. Glance through the first few pages preferably with photographs of well-known personalities. Prompt her with appropriate questions to enhance communication.

Special materials: an armchair and a daily newspaper.

Comments: note the length of time Betty pays attention and the amount of information she is able to share with you.

COMPLETED INDIVIDUAL PROFILE

Betty is used as an ongoing case study throughout the book. Here is her individual profile.

Name: Elizabeth

Surname: Brown

Prefers to be known as: Betty

Date of birth: 1920

Age: 80

Education: teaching diploma

Previous and current occupation(s): retired teacher

Previous and current leisure interests: retired rower, active member of the Women's Institute, keen on exercise

Important knowledge, values and beliefs: comes from a small supportive family; early days spent in China, married for 40 years, has one son, receives a pension, used to live in a semi-detached house, needs glasses for reading small print, wears a hearing aid

Likes and dislikes: likes people but dislikes noisy people

Important background information:

Over the last year or two, Betty has become easily confused and developed short-term memory loss that is getting progressively worse. She has given up housework. Before admission, there were a couple of times when her electric ring caught fire because she forgot to turn it off. Her son, Sam, had to check that she was appropriately dressed. She might occasionally use the large plant pot as a toilet. Betty's friends found it difficult to understand her. Sam was also finding it stressful to cope with the needs of his mother at home. He wonders if his mother is depressed.

Betty has subsequently been admitted to a local care home. She has also been diagnosed with Alzheimer's disease and prescribed with Aricept.

Current challenges (based on individual's perceptions and results of assessments): is aware of forgetfulness

Current goals: to attend group orientation session on a daily basis with minimum prompting

Current strategies: to facilitate session for Betty and other residents.

Outcomes: (based on individual's perceptions and feedback from professionals) Betty will maintain her abilities for three months.

Exercise

Having studied the completed profile of Betty, choose an older person you work with and complete an individual profile using the same format as shown here.

CHAPTER 3

Communicating With Older People

What is communication?

Communication is an important part of human behaviour that involves the sending and receiving of information and signals to and from other people. It can be subdivided into verbal and non-verbal communication:

Verbal communication: this uses language, speech and writing. Speech can be affected by voice quality, emotion, intonation and stressing certain words, all of which transmit messages or codes about how we are feeling and the significance of the situation.

Non-verbal communication: this uses posture (body language), facial expressions and gestures, but not spoken language. Displaying and receiving non-verbal signals are an important part of interaction. When working with older people, verbal communication tends to be stressed however close attention should also be given to non-verbal signs. Non-verbal communication can be used to pass on signals about emotions, feelings, attitudes towards other people and situations and as an aid to verbal communication such as by nodding and smiling.

Argyle (1988) maintains that, while the spoken word is used for communicating information, non-verbal codes are used to establish and maintain interpersonal relationships. Argyle believes the five functions of non-verbal communication are to express emotions, to express interpersonal functions, to accentuate speech, to demonstrate personality and to perform rituals such as greetings.

Newson (2010) stresses that communication and interpersonal skills are often used interchangeably. However, interpersonal skills are different because they concentrate on self-awareness, attentive listening, observing people's reactions and sensitivity to the feelings of others. It could be argued that exhibiting sound interpersonal skills can make people more effective communicators.

Any form of communication needs to be clear so that people can understand each other. During communication it is important to think about what is being said, the importance of one's own body language and the messages being sent. At the same time, people also have to read or interpret the messages being received during the interaction with another person. Barnes (2003) suggests that successful interaction relies on rules, expectations and feedback received from others. Sometimes signals can be ambiguous and confusing. This may particularly be the case when working with older people whose means of sending such messages may be impaired in some way.

Selected literature in brief

The importance of communication in the good quality care of older people is illustrated by many studies. The 'Home from Home' report (Alzheimer's Society 2008) found that a 'typical person' in a care home spent two minutes interacting with staff or other residents within a six-hour period, not including time spent on care tasks. Harley *et al.* (2008) highlighted the importance of finding successful ways of communicating with people with dementia that do not assume that, because people do not communicate, they do not understand. Their research shows that people with dementia may retain more knowledge and understanding than they actually express. They found that the people with Alzheimer's disease in their study returned to language patterns learned early in their lives and referred to their own personal experience; this supports the use of life story work with people with dementia. See Chapter 10 for more information.

Caris-Verhallen, Kerkstra and Bensing (1999) observed the verbal and non-verbal interaction of nurses working with older people. They found that when nurses were short of time interaction was less about emotions, feelings and lifestyle and more related to the task at hand. They stressed the need for staff to be attuned to individual needs, and an older person's questions.

Factors affecting communication

Environmental conditions: the environment where communication occurs can be significant – furniture, temperature and noise level can all affect non-verbal codes and the behaviour of the people communicating. If a room is very noisy with facilitators rushing around, older people may feel that they are not going to be heard or listened to fully, and so may keep their communications short or not say anything at all because they feel they cannot or do not know how to interrupt. Physical space can also affect the way that non-verbal signals are received, such as the space between people when they are interacting.

Behaviour: the behaviour of people communicating during their interaction can also send messages. Looking away at the clock when in conversation, for example, sends a message that we are in a hurry and do not have time to listen.

Culture: non-verbal communication is learned and differs between cultural groups. Gestures can have different meanings within cultures and religions. In some religions, for example, there is a connection between touching and respect. How well you know a person can affect the way that you talk to them and the non-verbal signals used; you may joke with or touch a person you know well, whereas you would not do this with someone you have just met. Knocker (2002) suggested that some cultural groups are louder and more expressive in their usual communication and this should always be accounted for.

Age: some older people may not appreciate over-familiarity. They were brought up at a time when it was important to show respect and to address people by their full names rather than their first names. Establishing how a person prefers to be addressed and respecting their wishes can aid future communication with them. Changing attitudes can result in language changes, the introduction of new words and expressions, and different attitudes towards clothing and 'acceptable behaviour'. Some older people may not understand the expressions used by younger people or appreciate the way they behave.

Gender: we may use different types of words or gestures when talking to men than when talking to women. Some older people may prefer same-gender interaction and will not communicate as easily with a person of the opposite gender. Some men may not express themselves non-verbally in the same way as women, such as in the demonstration of emotion.

Clothing: non-verbal codes can also be communicated through clothing and hairstyles. Clothing can send messages about how we feel and how we see the occasion, and it is a means of expressing personal identity.

Case study: Residential setting

The official opening of a new residential home was being treated as a special event for and by the residents. A tea party had been organised in the courtyard, a celebrity was coming to perform the opening and residents had made an effort to put on their 'best clothes'. When the female celebrity arrived wearing jeans, there were many shocked expressions from residents. To the residents this was an important event – the opening of their new home – and it merited a certain dress code. Their interpretation of the celebrity's dress was that she did not see the occasion as very important. From the celebrity's point of view, she was following her signature dress code and wearing a 'trendy' outfit.

Medical conditions: any condition an older person has (such as failing eyesight, hearing or memory) may affect the way the person interacts and communicates. Parkinson's disease or a stroke may affect speech and movement. A 'mask-like' face or 'blank' expression may be a symptom of a condition such as Parkinson's or dementia and can affect responses. Some people may experience the loss of production or comprehension of language (aphasia). Others may experience word blindness, or the ability to communicate by writing may be lost (agraphia). When people cannot name an object but are able to identify it by touch, taste or smell, it is known as visual agnosia. Some people with dementia may experience reduced inhibitions that can affect their behaviour and communication with others. They may say or do things that other people find strange, unusual or out of character. During the early stages of dementia, people may struggle to recall words, names and details and become confused when trying to identify a person, even someone they know very well.

Visual and hearing impairment: people with sensory impairment may need additional information to help them, such as describing the room and layout to aid their orientation: 'There is a chair to your left, x feet away.' Introducing yourself and other people can help to identify who is speaking. Making sure that people can see your face, speaking clearly and facing people when talking to them can all aid good communication.

Case study: Jennifer

Jennifer has Parkinson's disease and her speech is now slow and laboured. When she is searching for a word, her eyes flicker. She will often say just one key word, which the person listening has to work with and fill in the communication gaps to find out more. Between each word there are long gaps of silence while she processes information and formulates her response, and 'conversations' with Jennifer are short because she tires very quickly.

Practical advice for communicating with older people

The following factors and approaches can aid communication with older people.

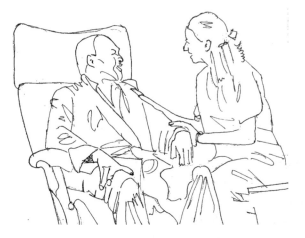

Physical aspects: make sure that people can see and hear you; sit at the same level rather than standing over them. Non-threatening eye contact and facing people who are talking so they know that you are listening to them is important. It is also essential to ensure that older people can see your face when you are replying. This may mean moving to face or mirror the person you are communicating with.

Body language: use open, positive body language and gestures and carefully consider the signals sent by the person you are interacting with. Certain factors may distract from the communication process: moving hands while speaking, or wearing dangling earrings or bold patterned clothing.

Facial expressions: smile, nod, respond positively and appropriately to what people are saying. While humour and laughter may remove threatening associations and aid communication, sometimes a smile may not be appropriate. It is important to be in tune with other people's emotions and to respond appropriately.

Patience: work at an individual's pace and give people time to answer; it may take a while for people to respond or they may tell you something you have heard many times before. Repeating information can be common for some people with memory loss. In this situation receive information as if it is the first time you have heard it.

Support and reassurance: consider whether it is appropriate to interrupt or contradict people. Sometimes reaffirming what has been said can encourage people to say more. Approach people in an open-minded way: you may be told something with which you do not agree. For the sake of harmonious relationships it is important to be tolerant and to listen to what people have to say. If a particular view is causing trouble with other group members, it may be possible to put forward an opposing argument so long as it is not done in a protagonistic way.

Giving and requesting information: keep sentences short and relevant where appropriate and do not overload people with too much information if this will tire them. Avoid giving people too many options and questions that they will find confusing. Too much information may be difficult to process. Similarly, some people may find a series of questions or double-meaning questions confusing: 'Would you like tea or coffee, do you take sugar, oh yes and would you like a biscuit?' can be broken down into a series of clearer questions.

Removing distractions: these could include turning off music and the television when people are communicating, and finding a quiet space for working where there will be few interruptions from other people.

Talking about yourself: sharing information is important to social interaction by breaking down barriers and aiding acceptance. Heathcote (2009) suggests that older people are more likely to trust people they feel they have something in common with. It is important to find an acceptable level of sharing and to ensure that you do not dominate conversations. Barnes (2003) suggests talking for as long as it works and not assuming that longer conversations are better than shorter ones.

Using interpreters: if working with people whose first language is not English or people who have reverted to their first language, it may be necessary to use an interpreter for one-to-one and group communication.

Asking questions

Asking the right questions is an important part of good communication. When communicating verbally a mixture of different types of questions can be used.

Closed questions: these elicit yes/no/don't know answers such as questions beginning with 'Do you...?' or 'Did you...?'

Open questions: these require older people to choose what they say and to offer more information, such as those starting with how, why, when, what, which, where, or 'Tell me about your...'

Statements: sometimes asking too many questions can be off-putting for an older person. Making an interesting statement that captures a person's attention and then waiting to see if it generates a response may prompt conversation: 'What an interesting photograph of your family...' The key to this approach is having the confidence to wait for the person to process the information and reply. The SPECAL® approach (SPECAL 2010) recommends that asking questions causes people to have to search for answers, which is particularly distressing if people have memory problems. Instead the approach advocates listening to what people say and observing them to find out information.

Good communication involves:

- ensuring a room is quiet and free from distractions

- putting people at ease by talking generally

- thinking about the way people are greeted and welcomed

- ascertaining how people would like to be addressed; some people do not like to be called by their first name. (One way to do this is to say, 'My name is… What would you like me to call you?')

- keeping questions short and easy to understand

- asking one question at a time, building up information as you interact

- using questions flexibly

- speaking clearly

- sharing information with people that may encourage them to talk to you.

Exercise: Communicating with an older person

Think about an older person whom you work with regularly where communication can be problematic. Run through these questions: What are the communication problems this person has? How do facilitators address these? Are these approaches working successfully for you and for other members of staff? Could you and other facilitators communicate with this person differently? Is there a particular communication tool that could be used to help?

Case study: Betty

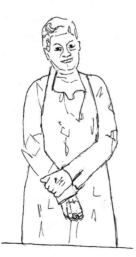

During Betty's stay in hospital when she was diagnosed with Alzheimer's disease, one of the nurses felt that she appeared quite lost as she repeated that she wanted to go home to 'see my mother'. She decided to engage with Betty and encouraged her to talk about her life experience years ago. Betty said that she had been a teacher and helped with the school choir. When the nurse asked Betty about the music she liked, Betty smiled and looked more alert.

Exercise: How to help Betty

Using the case study of Betty, consider what the nurse should now do for Betty. What messages do you think can be drawn from Betty's behaviour? What should the nursing staff do next?

Attentive listening skills

Listening to an older person is a crucial part of communication. Newson (2010) stressed that when listening attention should be given to the words spoken and the pace and emphasis of the words used. She suggests that we often use blocks to listening such as derailing: changing the subject because we do not like what we are hearing; advising; devising a plan of action before the person has finished talking; rehearsing; thinking about what you are going to say next rather than listening fully to the person; talking and judging; thinking to yourself that you would have dealt differently with something you are being told about.

LISTENING EXERCISES

The following exercises could be used for training purposes or to help you think about your own listening and interpretation skills.

Exercise: Reading the signs

In pairs, discuss words that express how you would feel if you wanted to tell someone something very important but you were unable to speak. Think of words to describe how you might feel if this was to happen to you. Words could be written on flipchart paper with markers. Consider such feelings as annoyance, impatience and frustration. Then discuss these feelings as a group and talk about how we can help people to communicate their messages if verbal communication is difficult.

Exercise: What's in a word?

In pairs, talk to your partners about a subject they can discuss easily such as a recent holiday or day trip. Everyone should take a turn in talking about this subject while their partners should ask them questions. Back in a group situation, ask everyone in turn to repeat something that their partner said to them. How easy or difficult was it to remember exactly what their partner had said? Next, use this exercise to discuss the factors affecting the way that we listen.

Communication using touch

Communication by using touch can include many behaviours, such as:

Touching another person: handshakes, a kiss or hug on greeting a person, patting a person on the shoulder to show support or friendship and touching a person's arm as a means of getting their attention are all forms of communication by touch. Touching can be differentiated: affective touch is a way of expressing affection while instrumental touch is used when carrying out a task. However, touch is culturally defined and interpretations of touch can differ: Wilkins and Mailoo (2010) point out that in the Hindu religion touching people above their shoulders or touching another person with your feet or shoes is considered disrespectful. Touch between genders may also be considered inappropriate in some cultural groups.

Touching one's own body: holding our arm, or stroking or scratching a part of our body can send messages about how we feel and our well-being, especially if accompanied by facial expressions. Together they may convey a message of discomfort or pain.

Negative touch: other forms of touch can send out negative messages about how we feel about ourselves, other people and situations. These include pulling, pushing, grabbing, kicking or tearing at something. When people send these signals, we need to look behind the behaviour to interpret the messages being sent. What has just happened? Is this a response to a recent happening or a sign of a state of well- or ill-being? Is the person expressing frustration, anger, fear or another emotion?

The communication of emotions

Sheard (2009) argues that feelings matter most in a person's life and that the communication of emotions and feelings are part of interaction. Behaviour regarded by some people as 'difficult' may be the way that older people are communicating their emotions, feelings and state of well- or ill-being. Such behaviours may include anger, frustration, aggression and withdrawal. It could also be a signal about how the people are dealing with their situation; unwillingness to do something may be a sign that people are feeling unwell, or that they do not want to be with a particular person. It is important that facilitators try to interpret this behaviour and work out what messages are being communicated.

Keene (2000) studied a range of behaviours from physical aggression to threats, verbal aggression, destructive behaviour and refusing to speak in a sample of older people with dementia. Verbal aggression was found to be the most commonly exhibited behaviour, amounting to 89 per cent of cases. When looking at possible causes for this behaviour, it was found that, for people with mild dementia, verbal aggression was more likely to be caused by frustration. However, in the later stages of dementia, all types of aggressive behaviour were more likely to be caused by intimate care that was perceived to be threatening.

Working with older people with verbal communication problems

Some older people may find verbal communication difficult or in some cases impossible. Coaten (2001) argues that we need to use 'creative alertness' when working with older people and especially people with memory problems. Older people may communicate aspects of themselves and we have to learn how to use the pieces of information that we receive and to celebrate the fragments of memory, thought and movement that may occur.

Case study: Stanley

Stanley had lost the ability to communicate verbally but still enjoyed attending the group reminiscence sessions at a residential home. He was known for his 'smiley eyes' that particularly 'lit up' when something captured his attention. The facilitator noticed that he liked the old local photographs, picking them up to study them closely. One photograph of a group of people at a local dance hall seemed to interest him particularly and his eye contact suggested that he recognised something or someone in the photograph.

Communicating creatively

Creative forms of non-verbal communication include:

Non-verbal signals: looking closely for an older person's non-verbal responses such as their facial expressions, eye contact and body posture can imply such messages as pleasure, recognition and like or dislike. See the case study of Stanley.

Pointing: people may be able to point to an answer or choice, such as something that is liked, or they may be able to respond to symbols or name cards. Memory prompts using old objects and photographs can elicit memory and communication (see Chapter 10 on reminiscence work).

Drawing and writing: it may be appropriate to ask a person to write or draw, thereby helping facilitators to identify messages.

Demonstrating: sometimes people may be able to show others what they mean by acting it out. In a craft activity, for example, they may be able to demonstrate without using any words how something was used or how a process was carried out.

Supporting equipment: it may be possible to use aids to augment communication – for example, ensuring a person's hearing aid is in full use, using magnifying glasses or large text and enlarging photographs for easier identification.

Communication tools: there are several tools on the market that can help facilitators communicate with older people. Examples of these are:

- flash cards and colour-coded picture cards such as 'Choices for Alzheimer's' (2009)

- 'Talking Mats': a communication tool using symbols on a mat that can be used to help people express opinions

- computers: assistive technology such as CIRCA (Computer Interactive Reminiscence and Conversation Aid) is a touch-screen computer system with images, sounds and archive footage to help people engage, reminisce and talk

- 'Pictures to Share' books: clear visual books that stimulate conversation and communication on different levels.

Dance, music, art and drama are increasingly being used with older people because they have the power to elicit spontaneous reactions and can be used to generate interaction between people. Creative communication allows people to participate in a different way:

Dance: people may not be able to tell you they enjoy a piece of music verbally; however, getting up and spontaneously dancing around the room suggests pleasure and interest (see Chapter 9).

Art: creating a piece of art is an expressive process. Colours and the way they are used can send messages about thoughts and feelings. Older people may also be able to express artistic appreciation, possibly with words or by pointing to paintings and art work that they like (see Chapter 7).

Music and singing: both these can be powerful ways of communicating. Some people may have limited verbal ability but can sing their answers; some people with short-term memory problems may recall the words of an old song; other people will enjoy making music by using percussion instruments (see Chapter 8).

Creative writing: older people may be able to use the written word to communicate their thoughts and ideas. Listening to poetry may inspire people to participate (see Chapter 12).

Hand massage: another form of tactile communication technique that facilitators can use with older people.

Always refer older people with communication difficulties to speech and language therapists.

Exercise: Making a communications charter

Facilitators could work with staff helpers to complete a communications charter for group and individual work. Here are two pledges to start:

1. I will think about my eye contact when I am communicating with people in the group and individually.

2. I will think about speaking clearly at all times.

3. . . . .

4. . . . .

Chapters 7–12 offer further information about creative activity when communicating with older people.

CHAPTER 4

The Importance of Using Assessment when Working with Older People

What is assessment?

The process of assessment is an important part of ensuring that intervention for the older person is appropriate and effective. Chapter 6 introduces the concept of the 'PIE' format, which comprises the process of planning, implementing and evaluating a group or individual activity. To appreciate where assessment fits within the context of working with older people, Figure 4.1 illustrates two additional steps that come before the PIE format can be used.

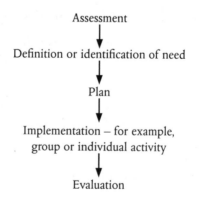

Assessment

↓

Definition or identification of need

↓

Plan

↓

Implementation – for example,
group or individual activity

↓

Evaluation

Figure 4.1: The place of assessment in intervention

Assessment has been defined as:

> ...the overall process of selecting and using multiple data-collection tools and various sources of information to inform decisions required to guide therapeutic intervention during the whole therapy process. Assessment involves interpreting information collected to make clinical decisions related to the needs of the person and the appropriateness and nature of therapy. (Laver Fawcett 2007, p.5)

Assessment, therefore, is a crucial step in the process of getting to know older people, in starting to value them as unique beings within the context of their lived experiences. It is important to remember that the focus should always be on the older person; this resonates with the concept of person-centred care that was introduced in Chapter 2. To progress this thinking further, consider the following reasons as to why assessments are carried out:

- To get to know the person you will be working with.
- To identify the person's strengths and weaknesses.
- To begin to establish which activities will be appropriate to use.
- To establish a baseline in terms of the person's ability to engage in the activity.
- To gauge the level at which the activity will be pitched.
- To monitor progress or lack of progress.

Hibberd and Chia (2007, p.284) stress the importance of 'thorough assessment and subsequent analysis of an individual's needs...' to ensure efficient use of resources. Without assessment there is the risk of asking people to engage in activities that may be inappropriate to their needs and which could lead to a number of consequences including the following.

- Refusal to join in any future activities.
- Complaints to staff, relatives or friends.
- Risk to health and safety and reduced well-being.

- Contraindications – for example, an activity such as throwing a ball may further damage a subluxed shoulder following a stroke; or, during a reminiscence activity, a particular memory may trigger heightened anxiety in someone who is suffering from this condition.

- Damage to the reputation of the organisation involved.

- Low morale – among both staff and older people.

Types of assessment

Assessments are categorised into two main streams – standardised and non-standardised assessments.

Standardised assessments

Standardised means 'made standard or uniform; …used without variation…' (Hopkins and Smith 1993, p.426). As can be seen from this definition, certain features need to be present before an assessment can be deemed standardised. Following extensive research and subsequent publication, standardised assessments will, according to Laver Fawcett:

- involve the collection of sufficient data for the purpose of the test (e.g. to screen for specific impairment)

- have established reliability so data are collected accurately

- use a systematic data-collection method

- have established validity so that data obtained are related to the stated purpose and focus of the test

- provide information about confidence intervals so the therapist can judge how likely it is that the test result has provided a true picture of the person's ability and/or deficits

- reduce the influence of bias or prejudice on test results

- have a record form for recording, analysing and communicating scores (Laver Fawcett 2007, p.152).

Non-standardised assessments

As stated in the following definition, non-standardised assessments, unlike standardised assessments, have not been through the process of rigorous testing in terms of reliability or validity: '...assessments that provide...information but have no precise comparison to a norm or a criterion' (Laver Fawcett 2007, p.154).

Some facilitators may not have access to or training to use standardised assessments and may therefore have to rely on non-standardised approaches to assessment. It is well documented in the literature that non-standardised assessments should be treated with caution (Laver Fawcett 2007) because they do not stand up to scrutiny in terms of providing valid and reliable measurements of a person's performance or abilities. This is not to say, however, that non-standardised assessments should not be used, because sometimes just observing or listening to people talking without the filter of a standardised assessment enables you to get an idea of how they function in relation to their daily tasks. A combination of both standardised and non-standardised assessments should prove beneficial for older people to gain an overall view of their strengths and weaknesses. Indeed, Prior and Duncan reinforce that: '...there is no standardised measure that can help a practitioner to understand what it means to a client to be affected by the illness or disability they themselves are experiencing' (Prior and Duncan 2009, p.88).

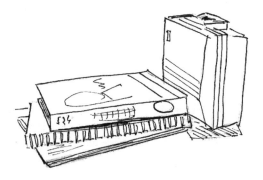

Table 4.1 lists some examples of assessments that may be helpful when working with an older person. Some of these assessments, however, cannot be used unless you have been trained specifically in

their use. Some assessments are specifically designed to be used by designated qualified healthcare professionals. It is worth enquiring if there are qualified healthcare professionals such as occupational therapists, clinical psychologists and neuropsychologists who have links to the setting in which you work, because you may be able to either borrow (depending upon your role) or observe them using a particular assessment tool with an older person.

Table 4.1: Commonly used assessments for older people

Title	Author	Characteristics
Abbreviated Mental Test	Hopkinson, H.M. (1972)	Screening tool to identify cognitive impairment in older people. Used to suggest that further testing is required depending upon results.
Canadian Occupational Performance Measure (COPM)	Law, M. *et al.* (2005)	Individualised measure to detect change in client's self-perception of occupational performance over time. Intended for use as an outcome measure as well as assessment.
Choices for Alzheimer's	Clairmont 2009 plc	Consists of three packs of colour-coded picture cards that help people to identify what they want to do, what they want to wear and what they want to eat. A person is asked to place the picture cards under the headings of 'I like' or 'I dislike'. The tool acts as a valuable means of communication to enable older people to communicate their likes and dislikes.
Dementia Care Mapping (DCM)	Bradford Dementia Group (School of Health Studies [2007])	Involves observations of care staff working with people with dementia. Results of observations are fed back to staff and recommendations are made to promote a person-centred care approach.
Interest Checklist UK	Heasman, D. and Salhortra, G. (2008)	Finds out information concerning a person's previous and current interests.

Title	Author	Characteristics
Mayers' Lifestyle Questionnaire (3)	Mayers, C. (2009)	Uses a person-centred approach to discover more about older people's priority needs and how these have an impact on their quality of life.
Mental Well-Being Checklist	National Mental Health Development Unit (NMHDU) (2010)	Provides a framework to help staff consider mental well-being. Consists of three evidence-based tables with prompts for well-being.
Mini Mental State Examination	Folstein, M.F., Folstein, S.E. and McHugh, P.R. (2008)	Screens cognitive function: provides measures of orientation, registration (immediate memory), short-term memory (but not long-term memory) as well as language functioning.
Quality of Life Profile: Seniors Version (QOLPSV)	Raphael, D., Renwick, R. and Brown, I. (1996)	Self-report measure examining people's perception of their quality of life in the domains of being, belonging and becoming. A person is asked to rate each item with subcategories for 'importance' and 'enjoyment'.
Rivermead Perceptual Assessment Battery	Whiting, S. *et al.*	Provides a preliminary assessment of a client's level of visual perceptual ability before therapy. Consists of 16 tests that include figure ground discrimination and body image.
The Pool Activity Level (PAL) Instrument for Occupational Profiling	Pool, J. (2008)	Used for people with cognitive impairment. Information is gathered and used to select appropriate occupations based on four activity levels: planned, exploratory, sensory and reflex.
The Residential Environment Impact Survey (REIS)	Fisher, A.G. *et al.* (2008)	Semi-structured assessment and consulting instrument designed to examine the environmental impact of community residential facilities on the residents. The REIS assesses how well a home is meeting the needs of the residents as a whole.

Given that there are many assessment tools available, consider the following questions, with accompanying rationale, which may assist in the process of selecting an appropriate tool. It may be that more than one assessment tool is required to assess different aspects of a person's functioning.

What is it you want to assess and why? (Consider what aspect of the person you want to assess – for example, physical, sensory, cognitive components.)

How are you going to do the assessment? (Consider the method you will use to conduct the assessment – for example, interviews, observation.)

Where are you going to do it? (Consider the environment you will be in when you are conducting the assessment. Is it appropriate? Is it in context?)

When are you going to do it? (Consider an appropriate day and time.)

Is the assessment tool available? (If not, are there resources to purchase it or can you borrow it from another care home or healthcare professional?)

Is the assessment tool easy to use? Are particular materials required? How long will the assessment take?

Are you able to make sense of and interpret the results? You will need to be able to justify why you have used the assessment and what it shows.

Will the assessment benefit the person you are working with? If so, in what way? Is it worth conducting the assessment? (Think about the resources required to do this. Can you justify it?)

Is the assessment tool used on a one-to-one basis or can it be applied using several group members simultaneously? (Consider how versatile the assessment tool is.)

If you are planning to do an assessment, are you trained to do so? (Some assessment tools require specialist training in order to gain access to the tools required – for example, 'Assessment of Motor and Process Skills' and 'Dementia Care Mapping'.)

Methods of assessment

As described in Table 4.1, some types of assessments dictate the method of assessment used – for example, the REIS consists of interviewing and observation. The following examples describe the different methods of assessment.

Information gathering: refer to the exercise 'Assessing a day in terms of quality of life' in Chapter 1 with the activity chart that records the activities that people engage in. This will give a useful indication as to whether older people are engaging in appropriate activities and also how much assistance they require from another person.

Interviews: this gives staff an opportunity to get to know older people and to begin to find out about their likes and dislikes. When interviewing, it is best to do so in a relaxed, informal manner, perhaps over a cup of tea or coffee. Remember that, depending upon the setting in which you work, you are seeking to build up a rapport so use this opportunity to have a conversation in a relaxed, informal environment that is comfortable for them. Refer to Chapter 3 on communication techniques; these are essential skills to use when conducting an interview for the purposes of getting to know someone.

Observation: there are many opportunities to observe older people carefully throughout the course of their daily living. Doing so will provide a means of assessing how they manage and function in everyday activities. It will also be a means of highlighting their strengths and weaknesses.

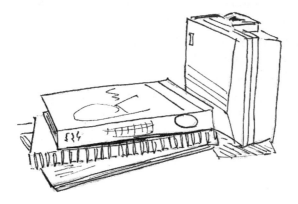

Reading through care plans, care notes and general documentation: this will give an idea of older people's previous history – both medical and personal – as well as how they are progressing in all aspects of their daily lives. Careful and regular documentation is essential for clear communication to enable all staff to chart people's progress, as well as for legal purposes.

Liaison with carers: some settings may have a key worker system or similar, and this will be an important source of information about how older people manage with their daily activities, as well as providing an insight into their general well-being.

Liaison with professional colleagues: this may include healthcare professionals who have an input into the care of an older person – for example, occupational therapist, social worker, nurse, general practitioner and psychiatrist. Understanding the purpose of a healthcare professional's visit and the conclusion or action plan to follow is a vital part of contributing to the overall assessment process.

Liaison with families and friends: it is likely that families and friends will know an older person well and may offer an insight into getting to know and recognise the person as an individual.

Implementing an assessment

It is important to plan for the assessment as far as you can. In the case of standardised assessments, this is essential because you need to ensure that you have the appropriate resources and materials with you. The environment may also need to be considered – where are you going to conduct the assessment and when? Sensitivity to older people's privacy and dignity is important. Are the clients aware that they are being assessed? Do they understand why they are being assessed and the implications of this? Do they need to wear or have with them any aids or equipment that they use, such as glasses, contact lenses, hearing aids, mobility aids and so on?

Case study: Betty

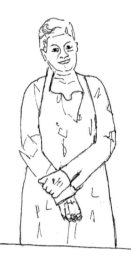

This case study illustrates how Ellen, a senior care worker in a residential home, uses different assessment methods to build up a profile of Betty. For Betty's full case study and profile, see Chapters 1 and 2.

Interviewing and information gathering: Ellen has been assigned the role of key worker for Betty, who has recently been moved from her own home to the residential home. To get to know Betty better, Ellen arranges to have a coffee and a chat with her in the conservatory of the home, which offers a relaxing environment to sit in. Before commencing this assessment, Ellen ensures that Betty is wearing her hearing aids; she is also careful to explain clearly why she is asking Betty some questions. Ellen starts off by asking Betty some open questions:

Where did you live?

Tell me about your family.

Where did you go to school?

What were your hobbies?

Where did you work?

Observation, information gathering, liaison with carers, liaison with professional colleagues, liaison with family: Ellen arranges to meet with some of the other staff within the home to find out how Betty has been managing with tasks such as getting in and out of bed, mobility, getting washed and dressed, toileting, feeding and so on. Ellen also organises a meeting with Betty's son, Sam, who visits on a regular basis, because she wants to talk to him about how Betty managed previously. She also arranges to meet with the psychiatrist when he comes to review Betty's medication and to assess her mental state.

Information gathering and observation: Ellen used a tool called 'Choices' with Betty. This consists of three packs of colour-coded picture cards that help people to identify what they want to do, what they want to wear and what they want to eat. People are asked to take the picture cards from each of the three categories and to place them by the 'I like' or 'I dislike' cards. Ellen then took a photograph of the completed work and placed it in Betty's care file for all staff to refer to. This tool acts as a valuable means of communication to enable older people to communicate their likes and dislikes; in addition, it contributes towards the concept of person-centred care (Choices for Alzheimer's 2009).

Reading through care notes, care plans and general documentation: Following Ellen's initial assessments with Betty, she added the information she had gleaned about her into a leaflet entitled 'This is me' (Alzheimer's Society 2010). This leaflet was designed by the Alzheimer's Society and includes a photograph of the older person plus information about their background, personal history and current needs in relation to different aspects of daily life – for example, communication, mobility and sleep. Some of the information from the 'Choices' assessment can be added within appropriate sections of the leaflet, such as likes and dislikes in relation to eating and drinking. In Betty's case, staff found it useful to refer back to the leaflet because it helped them get to know Betty and ensure that they met her needs.

Liaison with professional colleagues: The psychiatrist makes an onward referral to the occupational therapist who wants to conduct some standardised assessments. Ellen asks if she can be present during those assessments and the therapist agrees a time and date with Betty and Ellen in which to conduct them. The occupational therapist decides to conduct two assessments.

1. The COPM: this is appropriate for Betty because it will enable the occupational therapist to gauge her self-perception in occupational performance in terms of self-care, productivity and leisure. In doing so, this will help to formulate goals for intervention. If Betty experiences difficulty in using the rating scales, then a proxy such as a carer (Sam or Ellen) may respond on Betty's behalf.

2. The Mini Mental State Examination will be helpful as a screening test to assess Betty's cognitive abilities.

The DCM could be used with Betty to assess her state of well-being–ill-being, engagement and levels of interaction with other people and activity. However, using this assessment tool entails mandatory attendance at a course to be trained in its use.

Ellen found the process of observing the occupational therapist conduct assessments with Betty to be extremely interesting and she was able to learn more about how to assist Betty with her everyday activities. With the permission of Betty and the occupational therapist, Ellen passed this information on to the other carers working within her team so that they could all follow a consistent approach in their care for Betty.

By using assessment in this manner, Ellen and other care staff were able to find out which types and levels of intervention (activity, individual and/or group work) were most appropriate to Betty to meet her needs and aid her well-being.

Following Betty's assessments, the following recommendations were made:

- For all staff to communicate clearly when interacting with Betty.

- Use of individual work with an initial focus on encouraging Betty to engage in life skills (personal care activities) to maintain independence with washing and dressing.

- Participation in cognitive based group activities.

- To encourage Sam to attend a carers' support group.

Exercise

Consider what types of assessment you use in your place of work and why.

CHAPTER 5

Task Analysis
Working Step by Step

What is task analysis?

Task analysis is basically a process of breaking an activity down into its task sequence (Creek 2010). Creek and Bullock (2008) state that task analysis is designed to:

1. select a suitable activity to achieve an aim

2. help in the selection of a method of facilitating an activity

3. identify the sequence an older person may be having difficulty with

4. adapt an activity by changing it or reducing a sequence.

Task analysis helps facilitators in two ways: by giving them an awareness of the number of components involved in a task and enabling them to understand why an older individual is unable to complete an activity. It is a useful tool to support observations and implement individual and group work.

The following is an example of a task analysis:

Washing hands
Going to the sink
Putting in the plug
Turning on the cold tap
Turning on the hot tap
Turning off taps when sufficient water in the sink
Rinsing hands in the sink
Pressing liquid soap on hand
Rubbing palms and fingers together
Rubbing hands together, interlacing fingers

Rubbing palm and fingers of right hand over back and fingers
   of left hand

Rubbing palm and fingers of left hand over back and fingers of
   right hand

Rinsing hands in water

Pulling out plug

Using towel to dry hands

Essential factors

Peck and Hong (1994) suggest that, before any task is analysed, the
following factors should be considered:

- The individual's style of and capacity for learning.

- The speed at which the individual is capable of assimilating
  new information.

- The complexity of the task.

- Prerequisite skills that are necessary.

- The level of motivation that is necessary for success.

Different forms of task analysis

Hagedorn (2000) considers that a task analysis consists of a sequence
of self-contained stages or events with a purpose and product that
requires a maximum of about ten minutes to complete. She adds that
there are two forms of task analysis: content analysis and sequence
analysis. The following questions posed by Hagedorn (2000) will
help the process of task analysis:

What is to be done?

Who is involved in the task?

How is the task performed?

Where will it take place?

When will it be done?

Why is it to be done?

CONTENT ANALYSIS

For an example of a craft activity such as making a thumb pot, a content analysis is presented as follows:

>Purpose – to make a thumb pot
>
>Participant – one individual or a group of individuals who know how to make thumb pots or are interested in doing so
>
>Practical requirements – self-hardening clay, also known as air-drying clay, and sturdy table
>
>Location – clear space in sitting or dining room and adequate light
>
>Standard – completed thumb pot.

SEQUENCE ANALYSIS

However, a sequence analysis for making a thumb pot would involve the following:

Sequence and method

>Cut and wedge a piece of clay.
>
>Make the piece of clay into a smooth ball by turning it round the hands.
>
>Hold the ball of clay in the palm of one hand.
>
>Use the thumb of the other hand to press the clay inwards bit by bit towards the centre of the clay, turning it as you do.
>
>Repeat the process until the desired shape is reached.
>
>Make sure that the clay wall does not get too thin.

Exercise

Using the information in these examples, select an activity that you would like to use for an individual or group activity, and complete content and sequence analyses of the task. In what ways might completing such analyses be useful to your work in the future?

ACTIVITY ANALYSIS

In contrast to Hagedorn's content and sequence analyses, Hurtley and Wenborn (2000) suggest the following format for analysing an activity. It involves breaking the task down into five components:

1. Physical – for example, co-ordination and endurance.

2. Sensory – for example, vision and hearing.

3. Cognitive – for example, memory and problem solving.

4. Emotional – for example, internal drives and self-esteem.

5. Social – for example, relationships and interaction.

For example, if using Hurtley and Wenborn's work, making a thumb pot would involve some of the following aspects:

Physical
Wedging clay

Sensory
Feeling the clay

Cognitive
Understanding the concept of a round shape

Emotional
Reminiscing about childhood days

Social
If in a group, talking and anticipating the result

Making mango jam would involve some of the following aspects:

Physical
Removing skin of mangoes and cutting them into small pieces

Sensory
Feeling the skin of the mangoes

Cognitive
Following instructions

Emotional
Reminiscing about childhood days/cooking at home

Social

Sharing past experience

Exercise

Select an activity you would like to use within a group situation and analyse the activity using Hurtley and Wenborn's format. How do you feel this approach differs from the content and sequence analyses?

Here is an example of how to undertake a task analysis:

Name of individual: Jimmy

Activity: making a hot drink

Aim: Jimmy is following a programme to maintain and extend his skills in making a hot drink. He has some of the component skills but needs to link them with other parts of the task that he has not yet learned.

Equipment: mug, spoon, single packet of hot chocolate and a kettle of hot water

Done by worker	Done by worker and Jimmy together	Done by Jimmy
		Pick up a packet of hot chocolate, a mug and a spoon
Tear to open the packet		
		Pour powder into mug
	Pour hot water into mug	
		Stir hot chocolate
Pick up another packet, tear to open the packet, pour powder into mug followed by hot water		

Done by worker	Done by worker and Jimmy together	Done by Jimmy
	Place two mugs on a tray	
	Have a chat while sipping the hot chocolate	
	Wash spoons and mugs, tidy working surface and place empty packets in rubbish bin; dry mugs and spoons and put back in the cupboard.	

Exercise

Choose another familiar daily living activity. Complete a task analysis with an older person and check the level of support needed to complete the task. How can breaking a task down in this way be useful in understanding the needs of the older person you are working with?

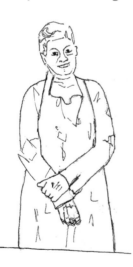

Here is an example of a task involving Betty. See p.29 for her full individual profile. Here she is joining a group activity.

Name of individual: Betty

Activity: baking muffins

Aim: Betty is following a programme to maintain and extend her skills in baking cakes. She has some of the component skills but needs to link them with other parts of the task that she has forgotten.

Equipment: recipe book, weighing scale, bowl, wooden spoon, baking tray, oven and ingredients: sugar, butter, flour and eggs

Done by worker	Done by worker and Betty together	Done by Betty
Preparing all ingredients	Reading the recipe	
	Weighing the ingredients	
		Sieving the flour
		Adding the flour, sugar, butter and eggs
		Stirring the mixture
	Beating the mixture	
		Greasing the baking tray
	Putting the mixture into the tray	
	Placing the tray in the oven	
		Washing up
	Having tea and enjoying the cakes	

Exercise

Use the example for Betty shown. Do you agree with the task analysis given Betty's individual profile? Now consider the following two statements. Why do you think these interventions would make it easier or more difficult for Betty?

1.   The task could be made easier for Betty by:

     (a)   You preparing the ready-mix cake mixture in advance

     (b)   Using a food processor.

Can you think of other ways to make the task easier?

2.   If Betty has a condition that might improve with regular activities, the task might be made more difficult for her.

Can you think of other ways to make the task more challenging?

Facilitation

Facilitator styles

As indicated earlier, task analysis will help a facilitator to select an appropriate method of teaching an activity. Methods may include the following.

Prompting: this is a frequently used technique to help individuals perform tasks by offering them various levels of support and encouragement. There are three types of prompt:

1.   A physical prompt is giving physical guidance given in varying degrees to help an individual complete a task – for example, demonstrating how to make cakes, and then giving help as appropriate while the task is being completed by the older person.

2.   A gestural prompt involves pointing to the ingredients to be used.

3.   A verbal prompt is in the form of clear and concise verbal instruction such as 'Cream the butter and sugar.'

Chaining: this is a useful technique because it allows complex tasks to be broken down into component parts and it constantly reinforces previously learned elements. To use chaining, the target task first has to be broken down into its component parts with the size, range and difficulty of each part varying according to the needs of the individual. Then, two methods of facilitating are available – forward and backward chaining. Forward chaining takes the component parts of the task and begins by facilitating the first stage. Once the first stage has been learned, the second stage is introduced and is practised along with the first stage; the same procedure happens with each subsequent component until the whole task has been taught. Backward chaining takes the same task and teaches the last stage first. Once this part has been learned, the previous stage is introduced and practised with the last component; this process is repeated until the whole task has been taught (Luebben and Royeen 2010; Peck and Hong 1994).

For example, baking cakes may involve the following stages.

- Switch on the oven (begin from here if you use forward chaining).

- Read the recipe.

- Weigh the ingredients.

- Cream the butter with the sugar.

- Sieve the flour.

- Add the eggs to the creamed mixture, a little at a time with flour.

- Beat the mixture.

- Grease a cake tin.

- Put the mixture into the cake tin.

- Bake the cake.

- Wash up all the utensils.

- Switch off the oven (begin from here if you use backward chaining).

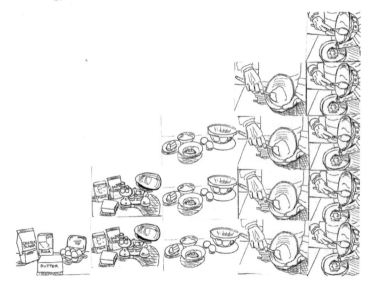

Task analysis may be used in a broader sense: take, for example, making and selling tomato chutney.

Growing tomatoes – buying seeds, compost and small pots, putting appropriate amounts of compost and seeds in each pot, watering them and putting them on a window sill.

Making chutneys – weighing tomatoes and sugar, washing and chopping the tomatoes, placing them in a container with the sugar, measuring and adding pickling vinegar, stirring the mixture until it is ready to be bottled, warming the jars, putting the mixture into jars and decorating the jars.

Selling chutneys at a fete – decorating the jars, pricing and placing them on a decorated table, greeting customers and selling them the chutneys.

Using chutneys to make sandwiches for sale – buttering slices of bread, slicing tomatoes thinly, placing them in the sandwiches and cutting the sandwiches into neat sizes.

Another method of implementing task analysis is through the work of Pool (2008), who has developed four activity levels to meet individual needs – for example, baking may be presented in the following way.

Planned activity level: use a recipe card to help an individual complete the task as much as possible without assistance. It is helpful for the individual to see a picture of the finished product (i.e. the cakes).

Exploratory activity level: ensure that the ingredients needed are familiar, and encourage the individual to complete specific tasks (e.g. to cream butter and sugar). Use the task as an opportunity for reminiscence.

Sensory activity level: ask the individual to put the butter and sugar in a bowl. Then cream them – either on your own or with the individual. Taste the mixture.

Reflex activity level: ensure that the individual is comfortable and can see what you are doing. Help the individual to complete some of the tasks (e.g. creaming the butter and sugar or sieving the flour). Enjoy the experience!

Questions for the facilitator

Physical: does the activity require or enhance hand-eye co-ordination and adequate posture? How can it be adapted?

Sensory: does the activity require or enhance sight and hearing? How can it be adapted?

Cognitive: does the activity require or enhance attention? Does the older person have clearly identified cognitive difficulties? How can the activity be adapted?

Emotional: does the activity enhance self-esteem? How can it be supported? Does the older person have challenging behaviour? How can this be minimised?

Social: does the activity require or enhance interaction? How can it be adapted?

Reinforcement

Another key component of the facilitating process with a group or individual is the use of an appropriate level of reinforcement. This could include genuine verbal compliments on completion of the task, or part of the task, a discussion group to talk about the process or a celebration of the end product such as eating the cake or displaying the work.

Chapter 6

Initiating and Creating a Group

What is a group?

According to Bender, Norris and Bauckham (1994), a group consists of individuals of all ages who are classed together because they share a purpose or need. Being a member of a group can serve many purposes depending on people's individual needs and situations – for example, cooking might be seen by some as a leisure activity but by others as an important life skill that gives them a measure of independence.

Resources needed to establish a group

To get a group started and running successfully, the following resources should be considered.

- Funding to establish the group.

- A space or venue for the group to meet.

- Staff support to maintain the group.

- Interested people to join the group.

FUNDING

In residential settings limited funding will be required to establish a group. When bringing people together to form a new group, as in the community, funding may be required for the venue, refreshments, equipment and transport. With carer support groups funding may also be needed for the provision of care for the cared-for member while carers attend the group. Funding could be sourced from the following:

- Small grants: a Directory of Grant Making Trusts or an online search will help to locate such organisations.

- Local and district government bodies may be willing to provide grant support for local group activity. Some grant-giving bodies ask for 'match funding' – that is, for you to provide money from another source. In some cases this can be in the form of 'in kind' assistance such as the hours put in by facilitators and volunteers.

- Sponsorship: from local companies, industries and banks, which may promote you as their organisation of the year.

- 'In kind' sponsorship: local organisations may provide, for example, a venue or meeting room free of charge, volunteers to help, refreshments for breaks or discounts on materials for crafts. Facilitators should consider other existing groups that could offer support.

- Subscription: group members could be asked to pay a fee for each session.

A MEETING PLACE

Finding a suitable meeting space should involve consideration of such factors as location, size of space required, the nature of the group activity, the type and size of equipment to be used, disabled access to the building and facilities within such as toilets and kitchen, lighting, seating, tables, parking and transport access. Consideration should also be given to how many people will be needed to set up the room (moving tables and chairs, for example) and pack away at the end of the session, and how long this will take.

The importance of the environment as an influencing factor in facilitating groups is reinforced by Robertson and Fitzgerald (2010) who acknowledge the 'interplay' between the physical and social environment in two residential homes. Certain aspects of the environment can be manipulated to create a variety of moods and atmospheres within groups, including the arrangement of rooms and seating patterns, room space and size, and colour, sound and light levels. These will now be considered in turn.

ARRANGEMENT OF ROOMS AND SEATING PATTERNS

The arrangement of tables, chairs and equipment within a room can significantly influence the way in which the room is used; this underlines the conceptual differences between work, social and recreational activities.

Work groups may need several high tables on which different activities can be carried out. In these instances, people are usually seated in upright chairs, while facilitators stand (or sit and move around the group regularly) reinforcing a supervisory relationship through the differences in posture.

Socially orientated groups are more likely to have low chairs in a circle or semicircle, and to have facilitators seated as group members, promoting greater feelings of equality and informality.

Recreational activities may dispense with seating arrangements altogether and, by having only a few chairs available at various points of the room, may encourage everyone to move, participate and mix with their colleagues.

ROOM SPACE AND SIZE

The size of a room and the space available are factors that can work either for or against the success of a group. Some groups cannot run without adequate space, while others benefit from the feeling of personal security and group identity that can be created by small, appropriately furnished rooms. Activities concerned with encouraging responses and interactions can be difficult to run in, for instance, a large, echoing games hall. If different sized rooms are not available, then screens or floor-to-ceiling curtains can be used to increase flexibility.

Case study: Familiar room

Two support workers, reminiscing with a small group of people with dementia, set up an afternoon tea session with old cups and saucers, cakes, doilies, etc. in a room upstairs not usually used for their sessions and which involved a trip in a lift. Despite extensive preparation by the facilitator to create an enjoyable group activity, the people with dementia were disorientated by working in a different setting, and kept asking to go back to the 'safety' of their usual reminiscing room.

COLOUR, SOUND AND LIGHT LEVELS

Colour, sound and light are powerful manipulators of the environment and can exert considerable influence on the mood or atmosphere of the group activity. Consider how you can utilise these factors according to the type of activity you are running – for example, if resources allow, choose a light, airy room with gentle music for relaxation-type activities.

SUPPORT STAFF TO MAINTAIN THE GROUP

Facilitators may need additional people to help them run and maintain a group. From the outset helpers and facilitators need to understand:

- the purpose of the group
- how the group will benefit its members
- their role in the group structure
- the level of commitment required – that is, what they will be required to do in order to keep the group running.

Certain approaches can be used by facilitators to keep support staff committed to and involved in the group. These include:

- involving all helpers in decision making regarding the group's activity
- using the particular skills of the helpers
- ensuring that helpers feel that they are playing a purposeful role
- addressing concerns that helpers have
- listening to what support helpers have to say about how they feel the group is being run
- regular debriefing and evaluation following group activity.

Group facilitator, roles and management

All facilitators need to be aware of the different roles they are expected to adopt. Faciltators must be able to command the attention of the group, and to move the group through the activity to the achievement of the goals of the group, but they cannot do this alone. Whatever role the facilitator adopts, the helpers within the group need to mirror and support this. It is important for the facilitator to be aware of what is happening within the group, to be constantly observing the dynamics and to respond appropriately as these evolve.

Facilitator can adopt differing roles to help influence the group dynamics. Indeed, these roles may be interchangeable depending upon the progress of the group and the needs of its members. For example, when the group commences, the facilitator may adopt the role of 'explainer', whereas if, during the course of the group, some of the members become disruptive, the facilitator may then need to slip into a 'controller' role. The following facilitator roles can be adopted:

Explainer: facilitators within a group are responsible for ensuring that group members understand what is required of them. This means being able to express ideas or instructions clearly and effectively (without being patronising), varying the tone, volume and cadence of the voice to emphasise the importance of various comments, and making effective use of non-verbal communication – for example, posture, gesture, signs and facial expression.

Encourager: group members need to be encouraged to participate and achieve as much as possible, and facilitators need to know how much encouragement each person needs (and when to give it).

Controller: any group needs to feel that those leading it are in control, and can deal with any disruptions that may occur. In addition to this, facilitators need to be able to manipulate the directions of the group to keep it close to planned teaching objectives, and to keep clients working towards individual goals.

Innovator: closed groups can be static in nature, so facilitators also need to be innovators. This need not necessarily involve developing new projects and activities, but it does require them to bring new experiences and ideas into the group.

Trainer: obviously anyone involved in group work needs to know why the group is running, what is to be achieved and how individuals are to work towards planned goals. In addition, facilitators should also be skilled in a range of teaching styles and techniques, and understand how to meet individual learning difficulties.

Observer: if group work aims are to be met, facilitators within the group must be able to observe and evaluate what happens, and keep appropriate records.

However, the most important requirement in effective group leadership is good communication between all facilitators. Close working relationships make everything much easier to achieve, and make the group experience more enjoyable.

Responding to different behaviours within the group

One of the challenges of group work is being faced with a range of different behaviours or responses from the people present. The facilitator and helpers need to be alert and sensitive to this in order to maintain group dynamics. The following lists some different types of behaviour with suggested responses that may be used to facilitate group dynamics to promote harmony within the group.

Dominating or over-talkative: acknowledge the person's contributions and suggest that others in the group should have the opportunity to contribute too. Ask the person to take responsibility for something (e.g. fetching materials, making a note to purchase something for the next time the group runs, etc.) to enable others to have an opportunity to participate.

Aggressive: ask the person to accompany you out of the room to assist with a task. Try and remove the person from the group situation to prevent an escalation of aggressive behaviour.

Anxious, shy or passive: gently encourage such people to engage in tasks that are within their remit so as not to pressurise them unduly. Try not to put them under the spotlight because this may heighten their sense of anxiety. Acknowledge and value any contributions they make.

Exercise

Can you think of any other behaviours and how you would respond to these?

Recruiting people to join the group

Potential group members could be identified in the following ways:

- Targeting an existing group of people such as sheltered housing residents or a lunch club.

- Advertising for members locally: in newspapers, libraries and doctor's surgeries, for example.

- Referral by doctors, social workers and charity workers.

- Word of mouth, by members suggesting another member.

- Continued publicity, in order to find both new members and ongoing financial support.

Group members must feel that attending the group will offer them something beneficial and that the group will meet their needs. The Nordic Campbell review (2008) suggested that a contributory factor to successful group-based intervention was that older people contributed to the planning and development of the activities. Giving ownership to group members and allowing them to make a contribution to the running of the group may help to maintain active ongoing support for the group. If people find that the group has lost its meaning for them, they are more likely to stop attending. Toseland and Rivas

(2005) believe that groups that offer some kind of 'reward' for being a member, such as resources, status and pride, are more attractive to older people. It may be possible that some groups can be 'enabled' by facilitators to become fully or largely self-supporting, with only occasional help from facilitators.

Organising a group within a residential setting

The following approaches could help you and other facilitators wanting to establish groups in residential settings.

1. Talk to residents and get their support. You could do this in a number of ways – for example, by asking for a slot on the agenda during a residents' meeting in addition to talking to residents on a one-to-one basis. You could distribute a questionnaire to canvas opinions on what residents think about group activities.

2. Speak to relatives and families and elicit their support and approval. Ensure that they understand what the group will do. It is possible that they may be able to help or join in with group activity. The *Home From Home Report* (2008) found that 54 per cent of families felt that their relative did not have enough to do in a residential care home. Some care homes are forming:

   (a) Relatives' groups, which give relatives the opportunity to come together in a group situation to discuss their concerns and worries about their family member in care. The development of new groups for residents and eliciting relatives' support for these groups could be discussed at these meetings. There is more information about carer support in Chapter 13.

   (b) Drop-in groups, sometimes using a café-style approach, where residents can take their relatives and visitors for tea and cake just as they would if visiting a café in the community.

3. Gain the support of staff both to encourage residents to join the group and to help with the running of it. Staff also need to understand the purpose of the group, and how the group can help them to deliver meaningful care.

4. Advertise the group using posters in the home or by including a piece about the group in the home's newsletter.

Case study: Pat

Pat is 83 years old and recently came into the residential home. She worked in a shop for all her working life. After having her family, she returned to be a shop assistant and was soon promoted to shop manager. Pat is therefore very well known in the locality. She lost confidence following a series of falls in her own home and her family were worried that she was not able to take care of herself. Pat was very reluctant to go into a home: she missed her pet cat, now being cared for by her family, and her neighbour whom she visited every afternoon for a cup of tea and a chat. Since her arrival in the home she has been in very low spirits and is reluctant to leave her room. The support staff feel that attending an activity group in the lounge might help her to integrate with the other residents.

Exercise 1: Working with Pat

Discuss Pat's situation and possible options to help her integrate with other residents. What type of group or individual activity might she like? How would you encourage her to join a group?

Exercise 2: Setting up a group

After reading this section, think about the process of establishing a new group from scratch. Make a list of the questions that need to be considered and addressed, starting with 'What sort of group do I want to form?'

This exercise could be completed before you run a group with older people or meet with them to discuss the type of group they would like.

Creating a group

The creation of any group requires careful consideration in terms of planning and implementation. Chapter 4 discussed the process of assessment and how to ensure that a group activity is suitable for the proposed members. It is useful when planning a group to consider what the aims are and the anticipated benefits: this will then help to ensure a match between the people concerned and the actual activity.

Running a group

When working in a group, it is important to set all work in a structured way. Using the 'PIE' approach can help group facilitators:

Planning

Implementation

Evaluation

This approach will be used throughout subsequent practical chapters. A PIE template to help you can be found at the end of this chapter.

Planning

The content and duration of a group activity varies in relation to the ability level of the group members, the creative medium used and the facilitator:older person ratio. Planning is an important part of all group activity.

Aims

Aims and objectives provide statements about what a facilitator is trying to achieve. Facilitators running each group should interpret these aims and objectives into sessional plans. This means facilitators have to select certain aspects of the overall goals, and then form them into a plan of work for the individuals within the group.

Preparation

Preparation should, in effect, be the procedure for getting everything – for example, materials, visual aids and equipment – ready at the right time and in the right place. Preparation also includes the formulation of the group aims and objectives and session plans. The aims and objectives should be formally written down for reference, but sessional plans only need to be brief notes about the order of work, and activities to be used. The more experienced facilitators become, the briefer these preparatory notes can be, but plans should never be so inflexible that they cannot incorporate spontaneous developments into the session. If more than one person is running a group, then written aims and objectives and shared sessional planning are essential. Once the aims and objectives have been decided, the following points should also be considered:

If using materials, what type and amount do you need for the purposes of the activity?

Does any part of the activity, including materials used, have any implications for special safety or health precautions?

Will the group be made up of one major activity, or several smaller, interrelated activities, and, if so, how are these subsections to be related and presented?

Does any part of the activity require the group to be subdivided, and, if so, how will this be done?

How large should the group be, given the nature of the activity involved?

Is it possible to deal with larger numbers by forming subgroups within the larger group?

What will happen if you have more than the ideal number of people wanting to join the group?

What differences are there in gender, age, ability range, behaviour, culture, motivation and concentration among group members, and how do those affect the session plan?

Does any group member have additional management programmes or aspects of a care plan that have to be incorporated into the session, and, if so, how will this be managed?

How can the available facilitators be used to best advantage?

Is the environment suitable for the activity? If not, what changes can be made?

What equipment and materials are needed for the activity, and are they available?

What will be the running order of the group, and who will do what?

Implementation
Presentation

This is the time when facilitators within a group prepare the group members for the activity. This may involve positioning the older people, explaining what is required or setting goals. The result of this part of the activity should be older people who are motivated to work well, and who understand what is going to happen. Stimulation of interest and motivation can be achieved by:

- showing examples of what is to be produced, or achieved

- giving a verbal description of what is going to happen – for example, identifying the ingredients and processes involved in baking

- asking group members to describe themselves, their colleagues or any recent news or events

- stretching and limbering-up exercises, or massage

- discussing themes or general topics before investigating them further – for example, discussing what everyone is wearing before looking more closely at descriptive words and concepts associated with appearance and self-care.

Presentation and motivation should not be hurried and may require instructions, descriptions and concepts to be repeated until understood. Facilitators should be able to present the same information and instructions in a variety of ways, to ensure that everyone understands and is ready to participate in the activity.

Activity

This is the part of the group session when the group members work through the session plan to meet the objectives that have been set. If the session has been subdivided, then the various subsections should link together to form a cohesive whole. For example, in a keep-fit session, the links between subsections could be:

- warming-up exercises

- movement around the room, ending in each client picking up a hoop

- using the hoops for balance and floor exercises
- working in pairs using hoops
- races to put the hoops away
- relaxation.

Initially, achieving fluent, smoothly run groups can be hard work, but skill comes with experience and attention to planning. Group members should be encouraged to contribute ideas and information that can be incorporated into a session, and consequently facilitators running groups need to be confident of their own ability to deal with such contributions and with problem situations. Confidence also stems from anticipating what form potential problems are likely to take, and being prepared for them in advance.

One of the most common problems is running out of work, or finding that the work planned is either too easy or too hard for the group members. Downgrading or upgrading the activity enables the facilitator to tailor it to provide sufficient challenge. When planned activities take less time than envisaged, the solution depends on the type of medium that has been used.

Case study: A craft group

Two support workers in a residential home

Group: six residents

Location: residents' dining room, with tables and upright chairs

Activity: to engage older people in making an Easter card

Aims: Dexterity, fun, stimulation, conversation with others, to make a card that can be given to someone else.

Preparation: Finding a design, making a sample to show residents, finding and purchasing materials needed, finding some Easter-related music to play, organising refreshments for a break.

Outcomes: On the day an emergency occurred in the home part-way through the activity. One helper was called away to help. This left only one staff member to help six residents of varying levels of ability and at different stages of the card-making process.

Exercise

What would you do in this situation?

Ending the session

Like the presentation, the conclusion of the group session should be related to the actual teaching content. While the presentation interests, prepares and motivates group members to join in the work, the conclusion provides reinforcement for achievement, feedback on performance and consolidation of key learning outcomes. Examples of ways to conclude a group are:

- looking at each person's finished work, comparing it with the original example, and restating the materials and processes that were used to create it – this can be followed by displaying the finished work, if appropriate

- reviewing individual performance on the amount of progress that has been made with a project

- using quiet relaxing activities after physically strenuous sessions.

The conclusion should also include time for group members to clear away materials and equipment, or clean up any mess that has been made. Learning to take responsibility for tools, equipment and materials is an important part of any form of group work, and generally this part of the session should precede the formal conclusion. Tidying and clearing away not only reinforces desirable activity skills but also reinforces concepts of cooperation, responsibility and shared commitment.

Evaluation

After a session has been concluded, the facilitators involved need to review actual performance and achievements against the original session plan. This evaluation takes two forms.

1. Evaluation of each group member's performance. This need not be particularly detailed, but it does need to be sensitive enough to monitor changes and progress.

2. Evaluation of the performance of the facilitator in meeting the objectives. This is best carried out verbally, but it is possible to use a written checklist (see Figure 6.1).

Any method of evaluation should include questions such as the following.

How successful was the activity?

Were the session aims and objectives achieved?

Were there any problems? If so, how did you manage them?

Could you have managed these problems differently?

What was the outcome of the activity? Did people enjoy it or not?

Which parts of the activity were successful and not successful?

Did anything go wrong?

What, if anything, would improve the activity?

Do you need to alter the activity in any way before you repeat it?

Evaluation will be discussed in more detail in Chapter 14.

Figure 6.1 is a suggested template that will be useful when implementing the PIE format and will enable you to implement a plan of action and subsequent reflection. Completed templates could then be kept together in a file to help you with planning future activities.

Exercise

Using the template in Figure 6.1, complete the various sections to help you when you next run an activity. This can be used for either a group or an individual activity.

Preparation for activity
Planning Aims of session: • .... • .... • ....
Resources required: • .... • .... • ....

Implementation
Activity:
 	
• Introduction:
   ....
 	
• Main part:
   ....
 	
• Conclusion:
   ....

Any other considerations: ....
Evaluation Reflections: ....

Figure 6.1: A suggested PIE template

CHAPTER 7

How to Facilitate Art and Craft Activities with Groups and Individuals

What is an art and craft based group?

Art and craft are creative forms of self-expression and can provide a means of communication when individuals have poor verbal skills and difficulties in communicating emotion. Creativity through art and craft can bring a sense of satisfaction, achievement and possibly the opportunity to resolve issues through the expression of feelings and the production of a piece of work. The terms 'art' and 'craft' are used here in the widest sense to include creative making activities with some kind of end product. This could include working with a variety of materials such as paint, paper, wood, wool, textiles and clay. The art and craft activities chart will help with the identification of ideas that can be used when working with older people.

Art and craft work may involve increased dexterity and hand-to-eye co-ordination, the revisiting of previously used skills, decision making, exercising choice and expressing creativity in design and colour. It can also stimulate the senses of sight, touch and smell, and be an enjoyable activity that brings people together. Friendships can flourish when people are sitting, working together and sharing ideas. Truscott (2004) claims that creativity can 'feed the spirit', and that we all have the desire to be creative and express ourselves in some way. This can be particularly relevant for people who have short-term memory problems and are able to express themselves creatively.

Selected literature in brief

McLean (2004) suggested that the creativity associated with craft work has the power to help people concentrate and exchange ideas, and encourage positive thoughts.

Wenborn (2004) stated that engaging in arts based activities provides not only a feeling of satisfaction during the task itself but also a sense of achievement in the end result.

MacGregor and Driver (2005) found that an arts project benefited people with dementia and the staff working with them. People with dementia were given the opportunity to express all kinds of emotion through artistic work. The authors found that even the most reluctant people with dementia were tempted by the artistic activities to get involved themselves while the staff enjoyed working with people in a creative way.

From the older person's perspective

The process of creating something also involves participating in a meaningful and often sociable activity that can have an impact on well-being and encourage a sense of achievement. Art and craft work can encourage reminiscing and, by linking activities to seasons of the year, people may be orientated to the present. Older people in care settings, who can no longer visit shops to buy gifts, may find pleasure in giving what they make to their relatives and friends. Participating in an altruistic activity can be an important motivating factor. Cipriani *et al.* (2010) suggest that such meaningful occupation can increase feelings of autonomy, role performance and satisfaction, particularly if older people are residing in long-term care facilities.

There are many arts and crafts that can be used to suit the remaining skills and abilities a person has, such as threading beads, sorting material and holding wool skeins. All these can encourage involvement and engagement with others. Art and craft work for some older people can be an important part of a lifelong learning approach and can help to maintain alertness by presenting a new challenge and purpose. Revisiting old skills can also have a favourable impact on the self-esteem and well-being of an older person.

Case study: Jack

Jack, a retired carpenter, attended a day centre regularly and had been very withdrawn since the death of his wife. When a flower box-making project was introduced, Jack was inspired to help the other men in the group make and paint their boxes. The opportunity to use his many skills with wood and getting involved in something meaningful gave Jack a new sense of purpose generally. The men enjoyed talking about their jobs and the things they had made and there was much laughter during the flower box-making sessions.

From the facilitator's perspective

Engaging in an art and craft activity can be a talking point, a way of sharing information and working with an older person. In this way, a facilitator can find out more about older people, what they feel they can and cannot do, and what they may need help with. Creative projects can be used to assess a range of abilities such as motor, vision, hearing, perception, concentration, memory, and verbal and non-verbal skills. It may become apparent that some members of a group have a particular skill that could be used further; the person could become an advisor to the group, show others how to make things, contribute ideas to the group and help less able people with their work. One approach the facilitator could take is to enable the older person to take on this role.

Case study: Lily

Lily, who lived independently, appeared to be a capable and outgoing lady. Therefore the facilitator decided that Lily would be able to complete the set task with minimal help while she concentrated on supporting other less able people. However, during the session it became clear that Lily was struggling with a stage of the making process, not requesting help and consequently becoming agitated because she could not do what she felt she should be able to do. The facilitator quietly offered support for the stage that was causing concern and Lily was then able to complete the rest of the task on her own quite happily. During evaluation between facilitators after the session, it was noted that Lily might need additional help with some crafts to avoid future distress.

The importance of creative self-expression

Bearing in mind the premise established that art and craft can be an extremely important form of self-expression, facilitators should always aim to encourage such expression wherever possible. One option is an open group structure where older participants decide themselves on the medium to be used and how they will develop their work following their own designs, interests, feelings and strengths. In this sense the facilitator's role is purely one of enabling and encouragement. Some older people, however, will need more structure, encouragement and an element of instruction in order to produce a creative piece of work. Others may say they are 'not very artistic' when asked, and may need the opportunity to recognise their own potential skills and abilities.

The importance of art appreciation

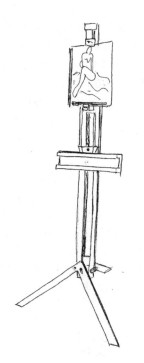

Halpern *et al.* (2008) compared preferences for different styles of painting displayed on postcards between people with dementia and people without. It was found that, although the dementia group did not have memory of the paintings, both groups showed the 'same stability in terms of preferential judgement'. The conclusion of this study was that care givers should be encouraged to engage in art appreciation with people with dementia.

The art and craft activities chart is a basic guide and by no means complete. It is not intended to be prescriptive or comprehensive – rather it is a starting point for facilitators from which ideas can be developed.

Art and craft activity chart

Working with paint and pencil	Drawing Sketching Painting in a variety of mediums Colouring Printing and stamping Marbling Using scraper board Art appreciation Life drawing
Working with textiles	Making a rag or braided rugs and mats Sewing activities: cushions, home furnishings, tapestry Felt work Weaving Making and decorating hats for occasions Stencilling on fabric Sewing a section for a wall hanging Patchwork and quilting Embroidery Making and designing home furnishings
Working with wool	Knitting squares for blankets and throws Knitting scarves Crochet work Bobbin knitting Making pom poms and animals Weaving Tapestry
Working with paper or card	Card making for occasions Making calendars, bookmarks, boxes and gift bags Making life story books (see Chapter 10) Scrap booking Making paper chains and lanterns Collage work Decoupage Papier mâché Origami
Working with other materials	Wood turning Woodwork: garden boxes for plants, bird boxes Salt dough modelling Clay modelling and pottery Basket making Glass painting Candle making Mosaics

Planning

Art and craft activity that involves a creative making process demands a high degree of organisation and planning. Wenborn (2003a) emphasises the importance of finding an appropriate activity for a person or group. This involves:

- assessing the person or group in terms of interests, abilities and limitations

- analysing what skills and level of strength the craft activity requires.

Consultation with the people participating about what they would like to do and the skills they would like to learn could also direct the activity chosen. Self-expression should always be encouraged. It may be necessary to gently encourage people who feel that they will not be able to undertake the task. McLean (2004) recommends the importance of not stressing the end product at the expense of the process from which older people may get enjoyment. Encouraging people to watch may lead to participation later, because they feel motivated that the task is within their grasp.

Knocker (2007) stresses the importance of ensuring that activities are appropriate to a person's cultural and class background. With craft work it is also important that the task is regarded as appropriate in terms of the person's age and interests. Zoutewelle-Morris (2010) recommends that, in order for an activity to be seen as relevant to an older person, emphasis should be placed on the use of good-quality materials.

Case study: Irene

Irene was hesitant about the stencilling task and said she would prefer to sit with the group and watch. The facilitator moved around the group helping, advising and encouraging where appropriate. After a while, the facilitator noticed that Irene had taken some equipment and was setting up her stencil like the rest of the group. At the end of the session, Irene was asked if she would be watching the group the following week. She replied that she would be attending and would like to join in from the start.

When planning an art and craft session, it is important to consider the following.

Which art and craft should be used? (The art and craft activities chart can be used as a starting point.)

Is the activity appropriate?

What does the task involve? See Chapter 5 on task analysis.

Will the task need to be adapted so that everyone can complete it?

What level of briefing will facilitators and helpers require in order to help older people participating?

What materials will be required?

How, when and where will they be found?

What equipment will be needed?

Will special equipment be required for some people, such as large-handled, easy-to-hold paint brushes?

Do some sections need to be pre-prepared by facilitators so that the tasks can be completed?

Are templates needed?

Do they need to be enlarged to enable everyone to use them?

Are written instructions needed for each older person?

Will some people need additional support during the creative process?

How will this be provided?

How will people be shown the making process?

Is a demonstration model needed to show people what the finished product should look like?

What are the health and safety implications of the task set and equipment being used?

Preparing the room

Part of the planning process is ensuring that the room is suitable for the activity to be undertaken. It should provide enough space for tables, chairs and equipment, with room for facilitators to move around easily to help people. An appropriate level of light to complete the task is also important. Before the activity can start, the room needs to be set up, tables and chairs arranged, and equipment positioned within easy reach. Thought should also be given to the extra items that will be needed: cloths for spillages, paper towels, waste bins and a water supply for cleaning brushes.

More information about preparation can be found in Chapter 6.

Preparing equipment

Making sure that the facilitator has everything that will be needed to run the session and for the older people to carry out the task is essential to the success of the session and ultimately the level of enjoyment and satisfaction felt by those participating. Equipment should be checked before the session to ensure that it is working correctly.

Implementation

The actual running of a session involving a creative process where a level of instruction is involved can take several forms. A starting point could be to tell people what the task is and show some examples of work that can act as motivators and models for practice. The level of demonstration needed will depend on the skills of the people in the group. It is important that facilitators consider how the activity will be done so that participants can see clearly and understand what they need to do. Some older people will be able to watch the whole making process and then proceed at their own pace with help. For others it is important to break a making activity down into steps or stages with a demonstration for each step and everyone working through it together. Facilitators can then move from person to person providing help, advice, support and verbal encouragement. Such decisions will depend on the older people involved, their levels of skill and ability and also the type of creative work. Some creative art and craft activities require people to work at their own pace and are not divided easily into stages.

The following pointers can aid the process:

- Facilitators should assess the level of help needed. Some older people may experience difficulty in using equipment or completing all parts of a task. It is important that the person is aided but that the task is not taken over by the facilitator. See Chapter 4 on assessment.

- The mood should be relaxed so that people do not feel pressurised by the making process or daunted by being left behind and not finishing.

- Unless the process is ongoing, it is important that the task can be completed within the time limits of the session so that everyone feels they have achieved something.

- In a session where free self-expression is being encouraged, facilitators need to consider how they will inspire people to think creatively and start their work. This could involve listening to music, reading poetry, looking at artistic pieces or visiting a gallery.

Case study: Sheltered housing craft group

A small group of female residents regularly attended a craft group and particularly enjoyed designing and making their own cards to send to relatives. Working on an Easter theme, the facilitator brought a large selection of good-quality card and materials and three sample cards with simple, easy-to-copy designs that she had made as models. She showed the group how to make the three designs and then let each group member decide what they would like to make. Working at their own pace, the residents made at least three cards each. Some were copies of the model cards, but many were individual designs that had been inspired by the process and materials available. At the end of the session, residents commented how much they had enjoyed looking through 'all of the lovely materials' and choosing colours and textures for their cards.

Evaluation

Bowden and Lewthwaite (2009) recommend reflecting on the level of enjoyment and participation in a making activity experienced by both participants and facilitators. Their evaluation sheet also asks for suggestions for improvements from both participants and facilitators.

Wenborn (2003b) stresses the importance of asking older people what they enjoyed and valued about an activity. She suggests that facilitators should consider people's reactions during the activity – what they say, their body language and their reactions to the amount of dexterity and concentration needed – against their sense of achievement and well-being. Wenborn points out that some older people may feel that they have not performed as well as they used to. If this is the case, she suggests looking at which aspects of the process have been valued and then finding another activity that concentrates on those aspects.

Celebrating what people make

This can help people feel valued and add to their sense of achievement and well-being. Allowing time at the end of a session for a display of work with refreshments can provide an opportunity to celebrate people's work so they can see what has been achieved. Groups may also wish to consider formal exhibitions of work to which relatives and members of the public are invited.

Case study: Village art group

The facilitator of a group of older people living independently who met weekly to draw and paint was impressed by the standard of art work being produced and suggested a public exhibition in the local church. The older people each contributed three pieces of art work and took it in turns to open the exhibition to the public and to talk to visitors about their work.

Case study: Exhibition in a dementia unit

Staff in the dementia unit of a residential home organised an exhibition of residents' art and craft work in the foyer. Invitations were made and sent to relatives and friends for a formal morning opening of the exhibition. It was a very happy occasion. Residents helped serve tea and cake and were completely engaged for the whole time – talking, sharing, looking and eating cake!

How to get started with art and craft activities

Task 1: Papier mâché bead making (Mills 2010)

What does the task involve?

Creating, painting and threading papier mâché beads.

What is needed?

Old newspaper, bowl, flour and water, tray, knitting needle, acrylic paint, paper varnish, strong thread, plastic covering for table, cloths.

Instructions

Collect old newspapers and tear them into small pieces.

Put the newspaper pieces into a bowl.

Add one tablespoon of plain white flour and water so that the papers are covered.

Mix the water, paper and flour together. The resulting mixture should look like grey lumpy soup!

Take a handful of the mixture from the bowl and shape into round beads.

Leave the beads for a couple of days on a tray to dry.

When the beads have dried a little, make a hole through each one using a knitting needle.

Paint the beads with a design using acrylic paint.

Leave the beads to dry.

The beads can then be varnished with paper varnish.

Thread the beads onto strong cord to make your own jewellery.

What could you do next?

Necklaces and bracelets could be attached to card, placed in cellophane bags and given as gifts; the activity could be used to introduce people to other making activities such as clay modelling, pottery and salt dough. Other forms of recycling craft could be explored.

Task 2: Using watercolour pencils

What does the task involve?

Expressing creativity through art work and the use of colour.

What is needed?

Pencils, rubber, watercolour pencils, paper suitable for watercolour painting, small brushes, water, cloths, mount board frames, suitable objects to draw (such as leaves, shells, flowers, plants) book containing examples of watercolour paintings and music to provide inspiration.

Instructions

Hold a mount board in front of your eyes and look through it so that it acts as a frame. You can then draw what you can see inside the frame. Alternatively place the mount board on the table and put an item of your choice within the frame; the item can then be drawn.

Draw a rough outline in ordinary pencil.

Use the watercolour pencils to shade in areas of the picture.

Put a little water on a paint brush and gently apply to the watercoloured areas. Do not use too much water.

Gentle rubbing of the watercoloured areas will produce a 'washed' effect. Looking at examples of impressionist paintings from an art book will demonstrate this effect. The colours can be merged to get different effects.

Leave to dry.

What could you do next?

Art work could be attached to the mount board, framed and displayed in an exhibition of work. This could be an introduction to using watercolour paint and lead on to other creative art approaches using different mediums such as charcoal and oils.

Exercise

What challenges, if any, do you face in implementing art and craft activities within your place of work?

CHAPTER 8

How to Facilitate Music and Drama Activities with Groups and Individuals

What are music and drama based activities?

Music based activities that include singing can be used to maintain listening, create discussion, enhance reminiscence and stimulate movement. 'Singing for the brain' is a service provided by the Alzheimer's Society, which uses singing as a means to bring individuals together in a friendly and stimulating social environment. Even when short-term memories are hard to recollect, music is easier to retrieve for older people with dementia. For others, holding and playing an instrument gives them the opportunity to be 'in control' and offer a means of expression.

There are a number of organisations that employ professional musicians to work creatively with older people – for example, Music for Life and Lost Chord. Music for Life musicians use improvisation techniques to draw out self-expression and communication skills, an approach that can be particularly helpful when working with people with dementia. Lost Chord runs interactive musical sessions in Yorkshire and Nottinghamshire using dance, song and instruments.

Drama activities can include charades, movement, mime and improvisation, puppets and masks, text and story work. According to Jennings (1986), the main focuses in drama are creativity and expression; tasks; skills, learning and insight; self-awareness and change. In a creative and expressive group, individuals may be encouraged to focus on a performance such as a play or a summer pageant. Apart from giving creative and aesthetic enjoyment, a group of this nature provides stimulation, encouragement and a heightened experience of self. The work also increases an individual's confidence through development of the imagination, communication and cooperation. In a group that focuses on tasks, skills and learning, the behaviour and skills of day-to-day life can be practised through role-play. Group members can gain experience of decision making and negotiation, and begin to develop some independence and cooperation. Drama at a basic level can take the form of charades, which most individuals have played at a younger age. Overall, drama enables exploration of roles, maintenance of relationship skills, and opportunities for choice and decision within a safe environment.

There are a number of organisations that use drama to work creatively with older people. There are theatre companies, such as Ladder to the Moon that involve older people in taking on roles in their shows so that they are not a passive audience. This can give an older person the chance to be a 'star', sometimes only for a few seconds but sometimes for an entire performance.

Selected literature in brief

Some of the benefits have been identified by Cliff *et al.* (2008), who reviewed the available research evidence on the value of singing for well-being and health and identified that participants experienced the following: physical relaxation and release of tension, emotional release and reduction of feelings of stress, a sense of happiness, positive mood, a sense of greater personal, emotional and physical well-being, and an increased sense of arousal and energy.

Drumming can have powerful therapeutic effects. Bittman *et al.* (2001) showed that drumming has a value not only on a subjective level in relieving stress and promoting personal and social well-being, but also physiologically by affecting the stress hormone and immune system.

Hill (2005) reported the remarkable results of a music therapy project with individuals who had severe neurological conditions. Individuals who experienced involuntary movements as a result of Huntingdon's disease were able to gain greater control through participation in the project. The end result was a spectacular performance at a venue in Cambridge.

Chia *et al.* (2005) described the activities of a music group for individuals with dementia and their family carers to reminisce through sharing and creating music. They cited a case study:

> B was thrilled and said her mother had not played like that for several years. There was something so authentic in the rhythm and in her style of playing that we felt this was early memory actively connecting with the present.

Powell and O Keefe (2010) described the benefits music therapy had brought for residents, staff and families. They reported residents with high levels of feeling content, relaxed and engaged in expressive activity. In one comparative example of well-being using dementia care mapping (DCM), where the same resident had been mapped in daily life, there was an increase from 17 per cent to 60 per cent in verbal and non-verbal interaction.

Roundabout (2007) reported soft positive outcomes for group members who had attended a series of drama therapy sessions. The results included increased well-being, a greater sense of connectedness, better self-esteem, an increased ability to communicate and a sense of being valued. At the beginning, members would often be disorientated, inarticulate and low in mood; at the end of the session, members appeared to be more animated, focused and far more able to articulate their feelings, thoughts and opinions.

Spelthorne Borough Council (2008) embarked on a project through the local strategic partnership. This was to encourage community cohesion by promoting good relations between young and older residents. It aimed to change perceptions and enable both young and old to develop new skills by means of drama. It was concluded that the project was a brilliant way of bringing two generations together and 'showing them that they are not that different from each other after all'.

From the older person's perspective

Wenborn (2003) said that engaging in music and drama based activities provides a feeling of satisfaction and a sense of achievement. For instance, individuals who are familiar with some of the sounds or songs may reminisce about the first time they danced or could be orientated to the 'here and now' by linking the activities to the season – for example, by singing appropriate religious songs such as carols at Christmas. Some older people may enjoy charades or the social aspect of attending a play. All these activities imply interaction with others and engagement with day-to-day activities.

From the facilitator's perspective

Engaging with older people in music and drama can be an important way of getting to know them. These are very 'sociable' forms of activity, which can bring people together and break down barriers. Facilitators can learn more about the older people they are working with. It may be that an older person has a particular talent – for example, in ballroom dancing – which can provide an opportunity to share skills and ideas with others in the group. In other cases, older people who lack confidence may need careful and sensitive encouragement.

Case study: Philip and Sarah

Philip has been very withdrawn since his diagnosis of dementia and his partner Sarah struggles to find things for them to do together that he will enjoy. Philip used to be very sociable but now is reluctant to go out. He becomes very confused and gets frustrated and agitated when he can't remember things he feels he should know. Sarah feels increasingly trapped. Friends suggested that they both attend as a couple a local singing and music group for people with memory problems. The group provides a friendly atmosphere and Sarah feels supported by other partners in a similar situation. Philip, who always enjoyed music, joins in with all the songs and his spirits are obviously lifted because he knows all the words.

The music and drama based activities charts will help to identify suitable activities.

Music based activities chart

Listening to music
Music appreciation
Singing
Participating in singalongs
Musical quizzes
Discussions
Playing with musical instruments and music making
Using selected music to enhance play reading, expression of self in painting, exercise, relaxation or reminiscence

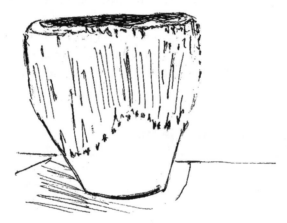

Drama based activities chart

Role play
Mime
Watching plays
Writing plays
Props making
Using drama to enhance movement and dance

Music based group activities – planning

An essential component is the identification of the older person's interests, strengths and limitations. Some of the assessments may include the following questions.

Is the older person known to have an interest in music and drama?

Is the older person able to move/sing/hold and play musical instruments?

How does the older person respond to the different types of stimulation in the environment such as music appreciation on radio and dramatic performance on television? (Munk-Madsen 2001)

What is the older person's level of activity? (Pool 2008)

It is good practice to involve older people in choosing music or songs. The preparation process should include asking the following questions.

Will it be individual or group work?

If individual work, where is the best place to do that? Unlike drama based groups, music based activities can be done on an individual basis.

Is there a spacious and quiet room for group work?

Who will attend?

What are the aims of the individual or group work?

What kind of activities and resources – for example, musical instruments – will be needed?

How will the session begin – for example, the use of a drum beat or a particular song to signal the start?

How will the session develop?

How will the session end – for example, with the use of soft music?

Will the activity need to be adapted so that all older people can complete the task, like padding the handles of some of the equipment such as maracas?

Will some individuals need additional support during the process?

How will this be tactfully provided?

What is the role of the facilitator?

Will helpers be needed? If so, how many, and what will their role be?

Preparing the room

An appropriate level of light to complete the task is important. Before the activity can start, the room needs to be set up with chairs arranged in a way that is appropriate. A semicircular arrangement may be suitable for music, but more space may be needed for activities that involve movement. Musical equipment should be arranged within easy reach. As music making can be noisy, it is best done in a soundproof room or in a place where other people will not be disturbed.

Preparing equipment

Make sure that the facilitator has access to musical instruments, CD player and electric socket that will be needed to run the session smoothly. These will create an ambience that will enable the older people to engage in the session with minimum interruption. Use of an old gramophone may help with reminiscence.

Implementation

There is no single format for running a music based group. A model that can be used for small group work is six to eight people with a facilitator and one or more helpers. This is particularly useful for music appreciation groups. Music-making groups may have a larger number of older people. Thought should be given to how the music based activity is introduced to the person or group. Is some form of demonstration needed to encourage and inspire people? A warm-up exercise may encourage more active participation. Thought should also be given as to how musical instruments are allocated according to people's choices, interests and skill levels.

Evaluation

Any evaluation of the work should consider the responses and feelings of the individuals taking part in the sessions (Munk-Madsen 2001) and the reactions and feelings of the facilitators about the whole process (Jennings 1986).

The following questions need to be addressed.

Do the older people show pleasure when the music sessions begin?

Do they join in the sessions willingly or reluctantly?

Do they hold and play with the musical instruments?

Do they show interest in listening to music?

Do they show a preference for a particular style or piece of music?

Do they interact with others in the group? (Woods 1982)

To what extent were goals met? Should goals be reviewed? Was there a problem? What caused it? How it was solved? (Leary 1994)

Powell and O Keefe (2010) have suggested the use of DCM, a set of observational tools that has been used in formal dementia care settings. DCM involves intensive and in-depth observations over a number of hours of the lives of people with dementia living in care settings. DCM highlights areas of positive, innovative care practice and identifies areas where improvements can be made to the social care environment.

How to get started with music based activities

Task 1: Music making

What does the task involve?

Listening, copying sounds, using hands to play instruments.

What is needed?

A range of musical instruments and soft armchairs.

Instructions

Ask people to name themselves as they clap their hands.

Pass around a musical instrument. Copy the facilitators – that is, play like them and stop when they do. Play a few sounds and ask individuals to repeat them. Use speed and volume to maintain concentration and variety.

Encourage individuals to start making musical sounds and ask them to look at another individual to join the music making.

Encourage two individuals to communicate by using whatever musical instruments they have.

Make a sound and use one or two hands to move like the sound.

Listen to an instrument and the music that illustrates the sounds. Encourage conversation about musical experiences: Who went to music lessons? Who can play which instruments? Has anyone taken part in a music competition? Can anyone recall playing music for guests?

What could you do next?

You could link music and movement and make basic musical instruments.

Drama based group activities – planning

An essential component is the identification of an individual's interests, strengths and limitations. Some of the assessments may include the following questions.

Why choose drama rather than other skills or creative processes?

What emphasis will the group have? Will it focus on creativity, tasks or insight?

How will individuals be selected for the group?

How will the group relate to the overall workload of staff (Jennings 1986)?

What is the activity level (Pool 2008) of the older person?

In drama based activities, Jennings (1986) suggested that adequate time must be allowed for warming up or opening the activities, for development that involves the main work of the session and for a satisfactory and relaxed winding down.

The preparation process should include asking the following questions.

Is there a quiet room for the group work?

Who will attend?

What are the aims of the individual or group work?

What kind of resources, drama sheets or props will be needed?

How will the session begin – for example, simple mime games?

How will the session develop?

How will the session end – for example, the use of silence and soft music?

Will some of the materials need to be adapted so that all individuals can complete the task – for example, reading enlarged scripts?

Will some individuals need additional support during the process?

How will this be provided?

What is the role of the facilitator – for example, in handling sensitive issues?

Will helpers be needed? If so, how many, and what will their role be – for example, in working with the facilitators?

Preparing the room

Successful drama activities need spacious, light and flexible spaces, where tables, chairs and props can be arranged in different formats according to the nature of the activity. Attention should be given to the type of flooring if a lot of movement is involved, and it may be possible to find a room with a dedicated stage area and lighting box.

Preparing equipment

Drama props and resources should be organised and planned in advance. It may be necessary to hire costumes, collect hats, bags, feather boas and other props, or for the group to make their own.

If working in the community, people attending the group could be asked in advance to bring items with them.

Implementation

Drama groups can be run in a variety of ways because each situation, individual and group presents different needs and requirements. Smaller groups may be better for a miming-type activity, for example, whereas play acting may involve a larger group of people. Facilitators need to assess the situation and the number of helpers required. It may be preferable to have a small group because drama based sessions can sometimes evoke emotions. When working with people with dementia, it may be more appropriate to work with smaller groups that allow one-to-one opportunities. According to Jennings (1986) the ideal session length for a group of ten clients is 1½ hours.

When implementing drama activities, it is also important to think about how to inspire people so that everyone enjoys and gets something from the activity, how characters will be allocated and how props could be used.

Evaluation

Jennings (1986) provided a list of questions, which include:

What sort of records will be kept of individuals or group activities?

Will these be formal or informal? Will video or written notes be used?

What were your feelings about the session?

How do you monitor the processes in the session?

Other questions may include the following:

How can you encourage further creativity?

How can you best use the space you have available?

Roundabout (2007) pointed out that it is important to take into consideration the physical and sometimes mental frailty of clients, as well as their generation and their cognitive ability. The questions need to be meaningful in the here and now because of the dementia and confusion sometimes experienced by members. As a result, they devised questions that would fit into the familiar context of the session and used the established forms of verbal expression and language.

How to get started with drama based activities

Task 1: Positive self-esteem

What does the task involve?

Writing, thinking, expressing verbally and non-verbally and miming.

What is needed?

Felt-tip pens, papers, magazines.

Instructions

Write a list of the things the individual is good at.

Paint or draw an advertisement of the person.

Look back over the last week and ask the person:

What have you been doing?

How have you felt?

List the aspects of behaviour that the person likes and dislikes.

Mime the behaviours!

What could you do next?

You could participate in a series of self-esteem workshops.

Task 2: Play reading

Some older people may welcome the opportunity to participate in play reading. A session could be broken up into a series of plays with intervals for refreshments and music.

Plays are available in sets from local libraries, but they have to be ordered in advance. An intelligent choice of play is half the battle!

When choosing plays consider the length of play you require. One-act plays are probably long enough for the uninitiated.

Consider the number of characters. Avoid plays with many parts in them because they can create confusion.

Avoid plays where too much of the dramatic content is in action, where crowd scenes are important or where the action moves rapidly from one place to another.

Choose plays that individuals understand and like.

Task 3: Theatre acting

Some older people may welcome the opportunity to participate in taking parts in theatre acting. A session could be broken up into a series of plays with intervals for refreshments and music.

What does the task involve?

Thinking, expressing verbally and non-verbally and miming.

What is needed?

Suitable props.

Instructions

Introduce the play to the group – for example, *The Inspector General*.

Clarify the theme and give some hints as to the main dramatic elements of the play.

See which of your individuals would like to participate. Stress that they are only required to read – no acting or moving around is needed. There should be as many readers as there are parts in the play and one to read the stage directions.

Tell each reader the important points of their character and suggest what they may like to wear in order to help them assume the character.

A few other props are often helpful to create an atmosphere or sound effects, for example, sound of horses' hooves, bells, footsteps. Tape recordings of these could be made as a complementary activity. Commercially produced sound effects are available.

Seat readers in the best possible proximity to each other. Everyone should have a table for their script. Label each table with the name of the character. This helps the reader and other members of the cast. Perhaps the group would like to do the play again for an audience.

What could you do next?

You could attend plays at the local theatre and make props (e.g. hats in an art session) for future plays.

Case study: Betty

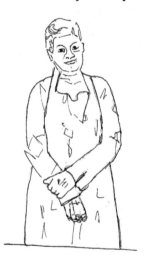

Betty recently had the opportunity to meet with some of the local school children and she was invited to recite her latest poem to them which they enjoyed hearing.

Exercise

What music and drama type activities might be suitable for Betty and why?

CHAPTER 9

How to Facilitate Movement and Relaxation with Groups and Individuals

What are movement based activities?

Movement based activities such as physical exercise and walks stimulate the brain and the body. They also help to alleviate tension and enhance interaction with others. They may also serve as a means of expression. Movement based activities can be adapted for older people who are immobile or use wheelchairs.

There are a number of organisations that are involved in providing movement and dance training for older people and their staff. Circle Dance offers simple and repetitive dance movements in a supportive circle combined with rhythmic music from all parts of the world. The emphasis of the session is on interaction and enjoyment. It is also a helpful approach for responding to the cultural diversity of service users. Other organisations that offer training include Jabadao, Vitalyz chair based exercise training, Extend, Medau Movement, and the Green Candle Dance Company.

Fit Together is a county-wide project originally developed by Lloyds Pharmacy and Active Norfolk to encourage a healthier lifestyle. The scheme is based on a national initiative established jointly in 2000 by Natural England and the British Heart Foundation, which aimed to get over a million people more physically active through brisk walking. The aim of the walks is to encourage and support people of all ages who are trying to increase their activity levels and lead a healthier lifestyle. Trained volunteers support walkers who may need help.

A physiotherapist is usually the best professional to offer advice on planning and monitoring exercise programmes for individuals or groups. Facilitators who intend to use movement and relaxation based activities are advised to attend a training course.

What is relaxation?

Every person experiences anxiety from time to time. It is a normal response when people feel that situations may threaten them. Anxiety can be helpful in certain situations when individuals need to perform well or cope with an emergency. Anxiety is often the body's response to stress, although some individuals may be more prone to anxiety than others. Anxiety symptoms are part of the fight-or-flight response; however, they may be considered a problem when the symptoms become severe and unpleasant and prevent people from doing what they want to do in their day-to-day activities. Relaxation can help such people to reduce tension and regain their ability to participate in daily activities. However, Heron (1996) has found that people who are forced to take part, or who experience intense distress or severe mental health difficulties, may not be suited to participating in relaxation.

Selected literature in brief

Older people should embrace a broader concept of health and physical activity that can range, for example, from walking, dancing and bowling to gardening and fishing. Most health benefits can be achieved from regular physical activity of moderate intensity (the equivalent of brisk walking at 3–4 miles an hour (5–6 km/h) for most healthy adults rather than formal exercise programmes. The social benefits of group exercise activities in later life should not be under-estimated in a population where social isolation and loneliness may be common (Andrews 2001).

Heymanson (2009) describes the benefits of circle dancing, which provide the opportunity to touch, hold, move together gently and be part of a group. Offering an activity that provides a shared togetherness, but which is not dependent on verbal exchange, is especially encouraging for individuals with dementia who find conversation difficult. It is also an enjoyable form of exercise.

Heron (1996) has listed some of the benefits of relaxation. These include:

- reduction in respiratory rate, heart rate, oxygen consumption and high blood pressure

- provision of coping skills that will enable people to manage in their day-to-day living.

Yu *et al.* (2007) examined the effects of relaxation therapy and exercise training on psychological outcomes and the disease-specific quality of life of older people who had had heart failure. While relaxation therapy was more effective in reducing psychological distress, with depression in particular, exercise therapy worked better to control fatigue symptoms. They concluded that relaxation therapy and exercise training are effective in improving the psychological and physical health of older people with heart failure.

In a ten-year systematic review with meta-analysis of relaxation training for anxiety, Manzoni *et al.* (2008) found that the results showed consistent and significant efficacy of relaxation in reducing anxiety. Treatments were equally effective in anxiety reduction, both for in-group and individual sessions.

From the older person's perspective

The process of participation in movement and relaxing activities can offer older people the opportunity to engage in sessions that offer a sense of well-being and health. The activities may be a source of enjoyment and interaction as well as engagement for some older people. They may also help to increase suppleness and maintain physical strength.

From the facilitator's perspective

Engaging in movement and relaxing activities can be a starting point for facilitators to understand the physical needs of older people. From group and individual work, the facilitator can find out more about what older people can do, their ability to participate in physical activity and where they need help. It may be that an older person has a particular talent such as being a retired keep-fit instructor or yoga teacher. Facilitators can also learn whether people would prefer the social occasion that a group movement based activity can provide or whether they would prefer the relaxation that an individual activity like hand massage might offer.

The movement and relaxation activities chart will help to identify suitable activities.

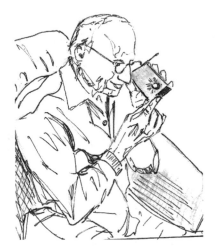

Movement and relaxation activities chart

Aromatherapy and hand massage
'Chill out' time – for admiring the trees, flowers, etc. within the environment
Dancing such as ballroom circle dance and foxtrots.
Diary time – set appropriate schedules for self-care, leisure and work
Exercise – active and passive examples?
Hobbies
Indoor games such as skittles and carpet bowls
Meditation
Multisensory environments
Music and movement
Outdoor games such as football, hockey, skittles
Use of the parachute to facilitate focused movement based activities
Tai Chi
Walking and rambling
Wii
Yoga

Planning

Movement and relaxation based groups require a careful assessment of the needs of the older person. The assessments in Chapter 4 can be used to identify the older person's needs in terms of interests, abilities and limitations. Some of the initial observations may include the following: Is the older person able to do the following? On their own? With the help of another person? With the help of two people?

- Rolling from stomach to back and vice versa.

- Moving from lying to sitting and from sitting to lying.

- Moving from sitting to standing and moving from standing to sitting.

- Standing.

- Walking without any equipment or with a frame or sticks.

- Walking and turning safely.

Payne (1997) said that, when dance is used as an art, it may focus on performance or exercise. According to Crichton and Greenland (1994), dance and movement give the body a voice and people an opportunity to learn about themselves and others. Although these concepts are for children, they are equally applicable to older people.

When planning a relaxation based session, the following questions need to be addressed by facilitators when they meet an older person.

Do you sometimes feel worried?

Do you sometimes feel uptight?

Does your mind sometimes jump from one thing to another?

Do you sometimes get thoughts such as 'I am finding it difficult to cope'?

Does your stomach sometimes churn?

Do you find that sometimes you can't sit and relax?

Preparing for the activity

For indoor activities, ensure that the room is spacious and safe for movement and/or relaxation. Some activities like dancing or using a parachute will require plenty of space for movement and possibly wheelchairs. Tables, chairs and other equipment should be placed on one side of the room. An appropriate level of lighting and curtains are essential for the sessions. It is also important that the flooring is suitable for the activity you are planning, such as a non-slip floor for dancing. Some rooms may have a dedicated dance floor if you are planning a tea dance, for example.

Some movement based activities may take place outside, such as yoga on the lawn or walking and rambling groups. People need to be aware of meeting places, how to get there, what they need to bring, such as waterproof clothing and a packed lunch, where to park and where the nearest facilities – toilets, café, etc. – are located.

Preparing equipment
Make sure that the facilitator has everything needed and that the older people know exactly what they need to wear (such as type of shoes and roomy clothing) and bring with them (towel or mat perhaps). Blankets, pillows and mats may need to be provided for relaxation activities. Maps may be needed for outdoor rambling. Music, a piano player or equipment for playing music, equipment for use of the Wii and refreshments for breaks all need to be planned in advance. These will ensure success and create a sense of enjoyment in the older people who participate in the sessions.

Implementation
The type of movement based activity will determine and present different needs and requirements.

Size of the group
Larger movement based groups like those for dancing will provide a more 'social' occasion whereas smaller groups such as those for armchair exercise may provide more opportunities for talking and discussion. When working with older people with movement difficulties, it is more appropriate to work with smaller groups that enable appropriate supervision and support.

Seating and arrangement of the group

This can be determined by the room size and shape, and the number of older people in the session. If it is a movement based group, then space should be provided for ease of movement. If it is a relaxation based session, there should be space for individual mats with pillows and blankets.

The following questions need to be addressed.

Will it be individual or group work?

Do you need music? If so, what type? Music player?

If individual work, where is the best place to do that? (A quiet space is needed for relaxation.)

Where will the group work take place? (A large space allowing ample movement is needed for movement based groups.)

Who will attend?

What are the aims of the individual or group work? For interaction? For exercise of the limbs?

What kind of activities and resources such as scarves, hoops, blankets and mats will be needed?

How will the session begin?

How will the session develop?

How will the session end?

Will it need to be adapted so that all older people can complete the task?

Will some individuals need additional support during the process?

How will this be provided?

What is the role of the facilitator?

Will helpers be needed? If so, how many, and what will be their role?

If working outside, how will people get outdoors? How many helpers will be needed? What resources will be required?

The following pointers can aid the process of implementation.

- Some older people may experience difficulty in completing some or all parts of the task, such as stretching shoulders when they have some pain. It is important that the individual is safely supported to complete the task and to guard against potential contraindications.

- The mood should be well paced and relaxed in the relaxation based session so that the older people do not feel pressurised by the process or the fear of being left behind by, for example, forgetting some of the steps. Ensure that the room is kept warm with soft lights and curtains drawn.

Movement based group – evaluation

Any evaluation of a session should consider the thoughts and feelings of the older people, in particular their ability to participate in the various movements, and the thoughts and feelings of the facilitators about the whole process.

Payne (1997) has produced an evaluation sheet for a dance movement therapy session. This covers the following.

- Time and length of session.

- Setting.

- Population.

- Props or music used and reasons why.

- Predominant themes – themes arrived with, themes evolving from group, what happened overall including structures used, responses and group dynamics, any changes noted, any specific expressions (verbal or non-verbal) assessment of socialisation skills related to objectives, objectives achieved.

- Future objectives for next session.

- Facilitator's own process recording.

Relaxation based group – evaluation

In her evaluation, Heron (1996) asked individuals to give a score of between 0 and 10 for each of the following components: physically relaxing, mentally relaxing and enjoyment of the technique – for example, progressive relaxation.

The following records may be useful documents for assessing an older person's level of engagement with the session.

Assessment of level of engagement by facilitator

Name of facilitator:
Name of individual:
Procedure: use the numbers 1–10 to note the older person's performance
Attention A little   1   2   3   4   5   6   7   8   9   10   A lot
Engagement (physically relaxing) A little   1   2   3   4   5   6   7   8   9   10   A lot
Engagement (mentally relaxing) A little   1   2   3   4   5   6   7   8   9   10   A lot
Engagement (enjoyment of the technique) A little   1   2   3   4   5   6   7   8   9   10   A lot
Thoughts and feelings about the older person's state of relaxation, strengths and potential areas for further development:

Assessment of level of engagement
by individual older person

Name of individual:
Name of facilitator:
Procedure: ask the older person to use the numbers 1–10 to note self-perception of performance
Attention A little   1   2   3   4   5   6   7   8   9   10   A lot
Engagement (physically relaxing) A little   1   2   3   4   5   6   7   8   9   10   A lot
Engagement (mentally relaxing) A little   1   2   3   4   5   6   7   8   9   10   A lot
Engagement (enjoyment of the technique) A little   1   2   3   4   5   6   7   8   9   10   A lot
Thoughts and feelings about state of relaxation, strengths and potential areas for further development:

How to get started with movement based activities

Task 1: Using a parachute

What does the task involve?

Working together to hold and move the parachute.

What is needed?

Parachute, ball, large room with furniture placed in one corner.

Instructions

Use a parachute that is made of bright colours with holding loops round the outer edge.

Encourage individuals to hold the loops and gently move them either slowly or quickly.

Place a ball in the centre of the parachute.

Encourage each individual to pass the ball round the parachute.

Try to bounce the ball.

As individuals wave the parachute, they could also sing a song.

What could you do next?

You could keep fit and visit Royal Air Force stations to watch demonstrations of the use of parachutes.

Task 2: Postcards

What does the task involve?

Thinking creatively, working together.

What is needed?

Postcards, possibly props.

Instructions

Ask everyone to say their name while moving a part of their body. Repeat this with a gentle movement and a soft voice.

Link hands to form a circle, to jump on the spot.

Let go of hands and shake arms and legs.

Stretch arms to reach for the sky or do pretend tasks such as picking fruits.

Touch a partner's hands and together, one leading, move hands and arms in whatever way the mood takes you. Work in fours, sixes and the whole group.

Use a theme to spark off individual creativity – for example, celebrations for the various New Years celebrated by the different racial or religious groups.

Bring a variety of postcards. Select one (e.g. a street scene) and get the group to portray the scene with the help of simple props. Invite some of the older people to take on the role of an ice-cream vendor who is touting for customers, some of whom may bargain for a large cone, etc.

Use soothing peaceful music to finish the session.

What could you do next?

You could visit the seaside or talk about day outings or long holidays such as a cruise.

Task 3: Relaxation

What does the task involve?

Lying down on a mat.

What is needed?

Quiet room, mat.

Instructions

Hands – clench first, let go.

Arms – bend your elbows and tense arms. Feel the tension especially in the upper arms, let go.

Neck – press your head back. Feel the tension. Bring head forward into a comfortable position.

Face – tighten the face by closing eyes tightly and clenching jaw. Feel the tension. Let go.

Chest – take a deep breath; hold it for a few seconds. Feel the tension. Let go.

Stomach – tense the muscle. Let go.

Buttocks – squeeze buttocks. Let go.

Legs – straighten legs and bend feet towards the face. Let go.

What could you do next?

You could take up a relaxing hobby, eat a well-balanced diet, take regular exercise.

Task 4: Do-it-yourself multisensory experience

What does the task involve?

Lying down on a mat or bean bag and enjoying the sensations.

What is needed?

Quiet room, mat or bean bag, lava lamps, soft music, hand cream.

Instructions

Invite the older people to choose between lying on mats or sitting in bean bags. Draw the curtains. Switch on the lava lamps and soft music. Pass the hand cream and ask them to massage the cream on their hands or each other, if they are comfortable with it. Ask them to watch the lights or listen to the music while they are lying down. Ask them if they would like to cover themselves with blankets. Finish off the session by switching on the light.

What could you do next?

You could go for a sauna, aromatherapy or massage, or sit on vibrating chairs.

Note: it is advisable to contact an aromatherapist for advice on massage and use of essential oils.

Exercise

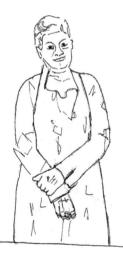

Betty enjoys walking in the garden and communing with nature. How could you facilitate this as a form of exercise for Betty?

CHAPTER 10

How to Facilitate Reminiscing with Groups and Individuals

What is a reminiscence group?

Reminiscence is the recall of memories, events and stories from a person's past. Our personal experiences and memories make us unique individuals. Recognising the individual and valuing a person's life experience and history underpins current care strategies, policies and approaches (for some examples, see Department of Health 2003, 2009; School of Health Studies 2010). Reminiscing is a vehicle for doing this: it is a powerful communication tool and a way of tapping into long-term memory, engaging with people and empowering them to tell their stories.

No matter what their age, people can reminisce; they remember different time periods, happenings and stories. Reminiscing can therefore be used in an intergenerational way to bring people of different ages together, and it is suited to both group and one-to-one work. Reminiscence is often viewed as an 'activity' to be carried out in a group setting. While this style of reminiscing can have many therapeutic benefits, reminiscence can also be used in one-to-one situations such as when delivering personal care or walking with an older person. In this way Heathcote (2009) suggests that reminiscing can underpin the whole caring approach. Not all people are suited to group reminiscing. This can be for several reasons: hearing difficulties, level of dementia, shyness, communication difficulties, depression, interpersonal dynamics, a reluctance to discuss one's life with others or purely because some people just do not like groups. Reminiscing can be rewarding for both the older person remembering and the facilitator who is listening. It can be an important contributory factor in building relationships between people, and it can also have an impact on well-being and future care plans.

Selected literature in brief

Reminiscing can have beneficial effects for individuals, people in group situations and the people working with them. Woods *et al.* (2005) found that people with dementia showed improved cognition, mood and general behaviour after reminiscing in groups. Moreover, family carers reported feeling a reduction in strain following the group sessions.

Chia and Hibberd (2009) studied the use of memory boxes, consisting of old objects and memory prompts from local museums, that were used by people with dementia, their family carers and support workers. They found that the boxes were successful tools, a way of encouraging people to talk together and, in the words of one support worker, a 'visual aid to communication'.

From the older person's perspective

Reminiscence work is a way of recognising people as outlined by Kitwood (1997) and acknowledging that they have something to say. Being listened to can increase the feeling of personhood, self-esteem and well-being. Older people will often remark that they have nothing to contribute, that they haven't done anything important. However, all memories are important because they are integral to the people concerned and their very being. See Chapter 1 for more information on person-centred care.

Case study: Ruby

Ruby lives independently and attends a lunch club several days a week. She listened quietly to the members of the group as they reminisced and suddenly became animated when the winter weather was discussed. She recalled arriving from the Caribbean to live in England as a young girl and seeing snow for the first time. Afterwards she remarked how delighted she was that someone wanted to hear her story.

From the facilitator's perspective

Facilitators can find out information about an older person that can promote understanding and help them to work appropriately in the future. Bonding with a person can therefore help them to do their job and add meaning to their role. Finding out about a person's life can help facilitators to see the 'real' person. More information about using assessment can be found in Chapter 4.

Planning

Reminiscence work can be used to achieve many aims and should not be undertaken merely for the sake of 'having a chat'. These aims could include:

- making someone smile after a recent illness

- providing companionship for someone who is lonely and living alone

- encouraging residents who rarely leave their rooms to interact with others in the home

- introducing a newcomer to the group

- helping a group of older people to integrate.

The first two aims could also be applied to individual reminiscing.

The importance of preparation

The preparation process should involve asking the right questions and deciding on action points:

Where will the group session take place?

Who will attend?

For individual work, where is the best place to do that?

What is the group going to do?

What is the role of the facilitator?

How will the confidentiality of memories be respected?

What care needs to be taken to avoid people getting upset by the recall process?

How will upsetting recollections be dealt with?

Will helpers be needed? If so, how many, and what will their role be?

How will the session start?

What resources, such as memory prompts, will be needed and where will they be sourced?

How will the room be arranged for a group session?

How will refreshments be included in the group or individual session?

The very nature of reminiscence work and the need to find memory prompts may demand that time is set aside to locate resources and think about how they can be used. Delegating duties to others can aid a busy facilitator.

Memory prompts

By touching the senses and providing a tactile, visual and audio experience, memory prompts can be used in group and individual work to aid the recall process. Holding an old object from the past can bring back memories of how and why that object was used. In addition to objects from the past, memory prompts can include old general photographs showing life years ago, personal photographs, old-style music, smells (carbolic soap, lavender, etc.) old film, newspapers, magazines, old-style clothing and examples of food that people may have eaten years ago. All prompts should be appropriate to the person, specifically:

- to their age: appropriate time periods for prompts are the 1940s and 1950s through to the 1960s, 1970s and 1980s for people at the younger end of the 'older person' spectrum

- to their gender: prompts should appeal to and empower both men and women

- to their ethnicity: thinking about the country where people were born and the time period when they came to this country is important because this will affect memories.

The memory prompts chart will help to identify prompts to use.

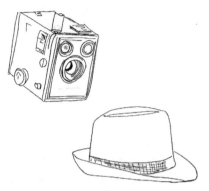

Memory prompts chart

Time period	Reminiscence prompts
1940s	Darning mushroom, handbag, trilby hat, carbolic soap, newspaper page, big band or Vera Lynn music.
1950s	1953 Coronation mug, coins, enamel dish, Bakelite door handle, Morris Minor car advert, rock 'n' roll or Elvis Presley music.
1960s	Photograph of beehive hairstyle, 1969 newspaper article 'Man Walks on the Moon', 1966 World Cup stamps, ten-shilling note, mini skirt, The Beatles or Sandie Shaw music.
1970s	Decimal coins, 1977 Silver Jubilee mug, platform shoes, Brut aftershave, pop music: David Essex, David Bowie, Bay City Rollers.
1980s	1981 Royal wedding item, 1989 newspaper article 'Collapse of the Berlin Wall', Walkman®, Live Aid music: Sting, Madonna.

Using memory prompts with older people

It is important that memory prompts are easily recognisable. People should be encouraged to engage with an item, by looking, touching, using and, if appropriate, smelling. This is particularly important if people have limited verbal skills or visual problems. Items should not just be identified or named but used in an empowering way to encourage people to talk or respond non-verbally. A mixture of questions and encouraging statements will prompt people to talk or respond in a non-verbal way such as pointing to an item or demonstrating how something was used. Non-verbal responses such as eye contact, recognition and smiling should also be encouraged.

Old-style music can be used in a variety of ways: to welcome people entering a room, for prompting discussion, as a subject for a quiz, for dancing (impromptu or planned), for movement and participation, to encourage singing and as a background during refreshment breaks. However, music played as a background during reminiscing can be distracting and can hinder people with hearing problems who may find it hard to distinguish between different sounds and noises in a room.

Case study: Bill and Diane

During a memories group for people living independently, Bill and Diane started to dance spontaneously, prompted by the music. Finishing to a round of applause from the rest of the group, Bill commented that the music was 'their song' – a tune they had danced to together many years ago.

Old photographs can also be an important talking point. Photographs of a well-known location years ago can encourage discussion about how times have changed. For people who find verbal communication difficult, other responses to photographs can be noted such as smiling and recognition.

Some people may be able to point to things or people they recognise. The most significant photographs are those belonging to an older person and facilitators should encourage their use. For people with memory problems, older photographs can be better prompts than more recent ones, which people may struggle to identify as their memory fades.

Old film can be used as a prompt for discussion. However, care should be taken that some people do not fall asleep.

Poetry reading can be an important memory prompt that can encourage discussion and active participation such as reciting poems together. It can also inform other activities including creative writing, drawing, painting or photography.

Where to find memory prompts

Memory prompts can be found in many ways: asking people for items, contacting museums and libraries which supply loan boxes and folders, and visiting antique centres, boot sales and charity shops. It is also possible to find memory prompts in specialist catalogues and on websites, especially buying and selling sites.

Implementation

There is no one format for running a reminiscence group. Each situation, individual and group presents different needs and requirements. However, there are useful pointers that can help a facilitator to reminisce with older people.

Size of the group

The larger the group, the more 'social' the occasion may be; the smaller the group, the more 'meaningful' the reminiscing experience may be. It is not always easy to encourage people to participate and talk in large groups. They may say less in large groups than in smaller, more informal settings or working one-to-one. In larger groups, people may become frustrated when others are talking and there is limited time for them to participate. A model for small group work is six to eight people with a facilitator and one or more helpers. When working with people with dementia, it may be more appropriate to work with smaller groups that allow one-to-one opportunities. Large groups, such as at day centres where many people may attend, could be subdivided into smaller subgroups with a helper joining each while the facilitator enables and oversees the whole session. After subgroup discussion, everyone could return to the large group to report back.

Seating and arrangement of the group

This can be determined by the room size and the type of chairs and tables available. Placing facilitators evenly around the group enables them to work with the older person sitting each side. Memory prompts can be placed on a table in the middle of the group and then passed around so that everyone has the opportunity to engage with them.

Case study: Group session in a residential home

Local museum outreach workers ran an afternoon tea and memories session for 16 residents. The room was arranged with four residents sitting around each of four tables. At each table, residents were helped by either a member of the museum team or a care worker. Each table was set out with a display of old afternoon tea items: cake plates, sugar tongs, doilies, recipe books and photographs. After a short quiz when residents were asked to recall different types of cake, all the memory prompts were used to encourage engagement and, where possible, discussion. The session ended with tea and cakes.

Refreshments

Refreshments, possibly themed with the session, can aid the recall process. Facilitators should decide on the most suitable time for refreshments, taking into account the nature of the session, whether old items that could be damaged are being used and the requirements of the people involved.

The importance of asking the right questions

Reminiscing involves asking questions, sharing information and listening. For more information about asking questions and communication refer to Chapter 3. The following examples may provide a starting point for reminiscing: 'Where did you live?' or 'I would like to hear about your first job...'

Some people may find a series of questions very threatening. A simple statement followed by a long pause can also be used to encourage people to reminisce. For example, when referring to a person's old photograph, stating, 'You look very handsome/stylish/pretty in that suit/dress...' and then waiting for a reply may prompt some interesting reactions and provide information to work with and find out more.

The importance of listening

Listening is discussed in Chapter 3. However, the following points are particularly relevant to listening when reminiscing.

- Showing interest and 'open' body language.

- Responding to memories appropriately.

- Reassuring people (they may be hesitant to tell their story).

- Being patient and giving people time to answer.

- Showing continued interest in a person's stories even if you have heard them before.

- Allowing time for everyone to say something if they want to in a group situation.

Tactics to use regarding upsetting memories

The confidentiality of everyone's story should be respected at all times and in a group it may be necessary to point out that people's memories should not be discussed outside the group setting. Reminiscence may involve talking about loss and upsetting episodes. Facilitators should aim to achieve an 'upbeat' tone from the start of any reminiscing, thereby sending a message that reminiscing is a non-threatening activity. Being told that they do not have to reveal anything they do not wish to can also reduce the chances of people getting upset. During the planning stage, facilitators should think about who they are working with and any known history. Potentially upsetting episodes should be avoided and themes for discussion chosen carefully to avoid possible upset. If the older people are not known to a facilitator, the choice of reminiscing subject becomes more significant and general subjects such as going dancing, sports and leisure, old cars, clothing years ago and going on holiday or days out could be a starting point. More personal areas could be avoided until the facilitator becomes more familiar with the older people and relationships of trust are established. If older people choose to talk about an upsetting episode in their lives without any prompting from the facilitator, it is because they feel able to do so.

If someone does become upset during the reminiscing process, this should not always be viewed as a problem. Showing emotions can be a cathartic process, especially if the older people do not have anyone else to share their stories with. Other members of the group may be able to identify with a person's story and offer support. Appropriate comfort should be offered and the upset acknowledged. It is important that the story and cause of upset are not dismissed because the facilitator and helpers are keen to change the subject. This acknowledgement should be given in a way that is appropriate to the situation, such as by asking the person to say more about it, giving time and listening fully to what the person wants to say. After listening to an upsetting story, facilitators could encourage the person to recall a happier story so that the reminiscing ends on a more positive note. The course of action to be taken after an upsetting story could be addressed later in the evaluation session with facilitators and helpers.

Length of reminiscing time

Each situation will present the need for varied approaches. Many older people welcome the opportunity to talk and will reminisce for some time. For others, a group session may come to a natural close. When people have short-term memory loss or find it difficult to maintain concentration, it is important that participants do not feel overloaded. Reminiscing could be divided into short slots with breaks for refreshments and appropriate activity, such as music and dancing.

Starting and ending reminiscence

An activity could be used to start a group reminiscence session to establish the theme or as an icebreaker. A very short quiz with questions about life years ago, identifying a piece of music, joining in with a song or a handling exercise are possible examples. A similar exercise could be used to end a session.

After the reminiscing

Reminiscence can generate many creative outcomes, and memories can be used to inform other activities such as art work, craft, making a display, making a life story book or a personal memory box, drama, poetry and creative writing. Chapters 7, 8, 11 and 12 provide ideas of how to develop these further.

MAKING A LIFE STORY BOOK

A life story book, a chronological record of a person's life and stories, illustrated where possible by copies of a person's photographs and mementoes, can be an important end product of the reminiscence process. Books can take many forms, including booklets, scrapbooks and folders, and their making can incorporate craft techniques. It is also possible to buy template books providing headings and suggestions for the stories and memories to be collected. Life story books value a person's history and experience. They can be important tools for future engagement especially if older people go into care, and they can ultimately become family heirlooms.

MAKING A PERSONAL MEMORY BOX

Heathcote (2009) describes personal memory boxes as collections of photographs and personal mementoes that have precious memories and stories attached to them. The purpose of a box is that each item can be used to encourage communication and engagement. Older people and their families can enjoy choosing the items to go in the box, and they can act as important memory prompts for the future.

Evaluation

Reminiscing is a learning process, a way of finding out more about people, and as a process it is one that is developed with practice. Evaluating reminiscence work by asking questions about responses, outcomes and achievements is valuable so that changes can be implemented, individual and group needs considered and progress made. Any evaluation of reminiscence work should consider the responses and feelings of the older people reminiscing and the reactions and feelings of the facilitators about the whole reminiscing process.

The reactions of participants to the reminiscence process could be evaluated by considering the noise level of the group, individual participation, body language and facial expressions. Taking into account the verbal reactions of group members is also important. These may be offered by participants without prompting or it may be necessary to ask for opinions. Reflecting on the session with all facilitators can provide additional feelings and reactions. If an older person recalled an upsetting episode from the past, it may be necessary to discuss how facilitators and staff should respond to this information in the future.

Case study: Khalid

Khalid facilitated a reminiscence session with a small group of frail older people. He felt that they had not enjoyed it as much as the facilitators had anticipated. The facilitators felt on reflection that the decision to move to a larger room with which the older people were not familiar had not been good. For the next session they returned to the smaller, more familiar room and everyone seemed much happier and more responsive.

The sharing of information between facilitators can be important, especially if older participants talked to one facilitator in particular. While it is important to respect the confidentiality of a person's stories and memories, some information can inform future engagement with that person, such as providing topics to discuss or not discuss. Thought should always be given to how this information is recorded, for example, in care plans.

If it is appropriate, facilitators could aim to enable the older people to take ownership of the group and/or the areas discussed. As confidence increases, group members may be able to participate more fully by bringing in their own memory prompts and choosing reminiscence themes, resulting in peer-led reminiscing.

Schweitzer and Bruce (2008) used a reminiscence evaluation form with participants, carers and volunteers who met for reminiscence sessions. They recommend asking questions about the level of enjoyment, things that surprised people, things they learned and friendships they made from the project.

Case study: Betty

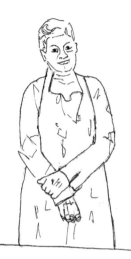

Betty has memory problems and experiences considerable confusion. Her long-term memory, however, is good. Betty lived in China as a child, did well at school, enjoyed rowing and became a teacher, working her adult life in a local primary school back in England. She was married for 40 years and had one son. Now complete the exercise below. A completed individual profile for Betty can be found in Chapter 2.

Exercise: Reminiscing with Betty

Using the information on Betty as a guide, how would you go about reminiscing with her? What would the starting point be? How could you work with Betty to produce a creative outcome from her stories and memories?

How to get started with reminiscing

Task 1: Personal objects and their memories

What does the task involve?

Working on the premise that everything can have a memory or story associated with it, including personal possessions.

What is needed?

Each older person, facilitator and helper brings an object that has a memory attached to it, which they are happy to recall and talk about in the group. They must also be willing for their item to be shown to the group.

Table and cloth for possible display, refreshments.

Instructions

Everyone, including the facilitator and helpers, has the opportunity to show their object or item and tell the story associated with it. People listening can then ask questions about it. You could make a display of all the items brought in so that everyone can look at and celebrate them.

Care should be taken with items that are particularly fragile and precious.

If facilitators feel that this will take up more than one session, you could ask half the group to bring something with them each time.

What could you do next?

This could lead on to further reminiscence work on the themes that have arisen during the session. You could prompt memories by borrowing a box of old objects from a local museum, visiting a local museum or getting some local history books and photographs from the local library, museum or archive centre. Creative outcomes could include making a life story book, a personal memory box, creative writing and depicting memories in a visual medium, such as art work, quilting and photography.

Task 2: Every photograph tells a story

What does the task involve?

Using people's photographs to empower them to tell their stories and help facilitators find out more about them. This can be adapted for group and individual work.

What is needed?

The older people are asked to provide an old photograph with a memory or story attached to it, that they do not mind recalling. Older photographs of a person's childhood and early adulthood may work more successfully than more recent photographs for people with memory problems. Facilitators could also bring in their own photographs and share their memories.

Instructions

Use the photograph as a prompt and starting point.

Encourage the older person to recall the memories and story behind the photograph. This could be done with carefully composed questions or by making a statement about the photograph and waiting for a reply. See 'The importance of asking the right questions' in this chapter and also Chapter 3.

What could you do next?

This could lead to making a life story book or personal memory box for the older person. A collage could be made using copies of photographs and written memories. For anything displayed publicly, the written permission of the older person and, if appropriate, their family will be required.

CHAPTER 11

How to Facilitate Life Skills Using Group and Individual Work within a Supported Living Setting

What is a life skills group?

Life skills constitute activities that are important to our survival as human beings. Within the context of this book, life skills can be divided into two main domains – personal and domestic activities. Personal life skills include personal care such as taking a bath, shower or strip wash, getting dressed or undressed, brushing teeth, hair care, applying make-up and keeping fit. Domestic life skills include preparing drinks or food, laundry and cleaning. Older people can sometimes neglect activities such as these for a number of reasons – for example, the effects of the ageing process or a change of role. Older people who no longer need to cook for the family or partners may lack motivation to cook meals for themselves. Simply being a resident in a home may also negate the need to actually cook. Maintaining life skills may be pursued through group work and/or on an individual basis depending upon the nature of the actual life skill and interest, the environmental setting and the needs of the older person.

Selected literature in brief

Warr, Butcher and Robertson (2004) report on the positive relationship between activity and life satisfaction in people aged between 50 and

74. Craig and Mountain (2007) discuss the creative opportunities that healthy nutrition affords and the positive influence on an older person's well-being of simple activities such as sharing tea and biscuits, laying the table, planning, preparing and consuming food. A study by Prosser and Staiger (2008), in which they introduced a visiting companion animal programme for older residents in a care facility, found that the exposure to animals resulted in increased social interactions. Wells (2007), after conducting a literature review on the benefits of dogs as companions and the positive influence these can have on people's well-being, cited the 'prophylactic and therapeutic' values that dogs bring.

From the older person's perspective

Being as independent as possible in an activity that is traditionally viewed as an essential skill for survival (such as self-care) can play a part in boosting self-esteem and promoting a feeling of pride. This in turn can give older people a sense of control over their appearance or perhaps the types of food consumed in terms of preparation methods or quantities presented. Living in a nursing or residential home, or being a recipient of a care package in a private or rented dwelling, may make some people prone to adopting institutionalised behaviour that in some instances can then become the norm. For example, if tea is made for a person, it is made by someone else; thus the element of choice is partly removed – for example, the cup is chosen, the strength of the beverage is predetermined and so on.

Case study: Richard

Richard, an activity co-ordinator, had been speaking to some of the older people residing in the care home where he worked who had expressed an interest in keeping some pets in the care home. At the next monthly meeting of staff, family and residents, the issue was raised again. The family of one of the residents said that they knew somebody who had some rabbits to give away. The family also said that they would make a donation to enable the home to purchase a rabbit hutch and run. Richard felt that rabbits were a good idea because they were the right sized animal to handle and sit on a resident's lap. The rabbits were a great talking point and some of the residents enjoyed helping Richard feed and look after them because this necessitated going outside to the courtyard area where the rabbits were housed. For the less able residents, every now and then Richard would clear the dining area, sit the residents in a circle and bring in the run that contained the rabbits so that the residents could watch them.

From the facilitator's perspective

For an older person who is able to engage in life skills, it can mean that the facilitator is able to adopt more of an enabling rather than a caring approach so that the older person becomes an active rather than a passive recipient of care. The facilitator will obviously need to gauge the level of assistance that the older person requires and this may vary according to the activity. It is important to be aware that there are different levels at which clients can participate in an activity; if not physically, then they may be able to indicate what clothing they wish to wear, for example.

The life skills activities chart will help to identify relevant activities.

Planning

The following points will assist in the planning of life skills-type activities.

- Assess all older people before engaging them in a life skills activity to ensure that it is appropriate for their needs and to determine their potential level of engagement. It may be appropriate to use the Mayers' Lifestyle Questionnaire (3) (Mayers 2009). In addition, see Chapter 4 on assessments.

- Consider what the likely benefits of the chosen life skill activity will be for the person.

- Consider the appropriateness of the setting or environment in which the life skill activity is to be carried out – for example, is it appropriate or realistic to do laundry activities within a day care facility?

Life skills activities chart

Self-care (personal)	Washing
	Dressing and undressing
	Hair care
	Brushing teeth
	Shaving
	Make-up
	Hand and nail care
Self-care (domestic)	Preparing drinks – hot and cold
	Preparing snacks – hot and cold
	Preparing meals – hot and cold
	Baking – bread, cakes
	Laundry – sorting clothes ready for washing (by machine or hand), machine or hand washing, hanging clothes in or outdoors for drying, ironing, folding clothes and putting items away
	Polishing shoes
	Mending clothes
	Cleaning, tidying up, sorting out
	Gardening
	Keeping a pet

- Does the life skill activity need to be carried out as an individual or group activity? It will be essential to do some activities on an individual basis – for example, getting washed or dressed when privacy is required to maintain dignity. With other activities such as baking, for example, it may be better to have increased numbers so as to promote group dynamics and thus enhance the social atmosphere.

- Look for opportunities to do one-to-one activities 'in the moment'. They do not have to be pre-planned so, for example, if facilitators are preparing the dining room for lunch and people wander in, you could ask them to help fold the napkins, or lay the tables.

- Does a risk assessment need to be completed before engaging an older person in life skills activities? If you are planning to work on a one-to-one basis and encouraging the person to be independent for part of the activity, is the person safe to be left alone? If doing heavy activities such as outdoor gardening, are there any contraindications (e.g. certain exercises are not compatible with certain health conditions)?

- Consider the timing of the activity – getting dressed at 2 p.m. is generally not considered the 'norm' unless there is a reason – for example, if someone prefers to rise after midday.

- Caution against having too many people in practical-type groups such as baking because individuals may require assistance and an environment such as a kitchen can be hazardous. Baking can be carried out in a number of different ways: examples are given later in this chapter under 'Implementation'.

- Consider the different levels at which someone can engage in an activity – for example, watching someone bake muffins and choosing the colour of the icing as opposed to weighing out the ingredients and mixing them together.

Case study: Tom

Tom, one of the residents with dementia, was recently admitted to the care home. He had been a farmer all his life and never married; therefore he was used to being self-sufficient. Every morning, when the care staff found that he had packed his bags thinking that he was returning home to his farm, they realised that they needed to give him a sense of purpose. The manager of the home purchased some overalls for Tom and got a name badge made up for him. Tom was then gently encouraged to work alongside the care home's maintenance man who made him responsible for looking after one of the courtyards in addition to giving him a shed to keep all his tools in. The staff also relocated his bedroom so that it was overlooking the courtyard. Tom never packed his bags again.

Preparing the room

Appropriate use of the environment is particularly important when carrying out life skills activities because, ideally, they need to be in context. For example, personal care activities should be done in the privacy of a person's bedroom, the bathroom or appropriate private room depending upon the setting. Similarly, where possible, kitchen-type activities are best suited in or near kitchen facilities. Think about the layout of the environment whether conducting group or one-to-one activities, and consider whether you need to have people seated round a table or to have several different tables – for example, if people are working simultaneously on different stages of an activity (preparing containers, potting up plants, watering, etc.) the latter type of layout enables the facilitator to move around the area, assisting where needed.

Preparing equipment

Ensure that you have all the required resources for the activity to run smoothly. For certain types of activity, it is important to use resources belonging to the older person to enable a sense of familiarity – for example, with personal care-type activities dressing people in their own clothes. For 'in the moment' activities, consider how appropriate it is for the person to be working alongside the facilitator and what materials will be used – if the activity is normally an institutional one such as pouring tea from a large teapot, is it appropriate for the older person to do the same? Some activities may require a risk assessment – for example, baking, which involves implements such as sharp knives, boiling hot water and hot ovens, all of which should be carefully considered and supervised.

Implementation

Personal self-care

One-to-one self-care activities can be carried out in the privacy of people's bedrooms. Facilitators need to enable them to do as much as they can for themselves. Consideration should be given as to whether people can be left alone for part of the activity, thus giving them a real sense of independence, or a facilitator could make the bed while a person is getting dressed. Encouraging people to participate as much as possible is important – even just choosing what to wear is a means of participation if they physically cannot help themselves. Refer to Chapter 5 on task analysis. This is ideal for using with a self-care activity because the different stages can be broken down into different components.

Domestic self-care

As mentioned earlier, this can be implemented in many different ways according to the needs of the person. Consider the following scenarios below:

Scenario 1: one-to-one activities for preparing cold drinks, snacks and meals are good for focusing on the needs of a person and encouraging independence. One-to-one work can also be used for the more anxious person in preparation for working in a group setting, or perhaps for someone who needs to experience a more challenging activity such as preparing a meal.

Scenario 2 shows how group-style activities can be used for making snacks or meals, then sitting down to eat together and clearing up afterwards – this is an important part of normalising the activity.

Scenario 2: this involves two to three people baking a cake or a batch of muffins. One person can weigh out the ingredients, another chop or prepare the ingredients and another stir the mixture or read out the recipe. While everyone is waiting for the cake or muffins to cook, the group members can lay the table for tea before making the tea and then looking at old baking implements and cookbooks or discussing how they used to bake years ago. The group participants can also be encouraged to wash and clear up on completion of the activity and to put items away.

Similar activities can be done in preparing a meal or making sandwiches. These can be organised around a particular theme – for example, a Spanish-themed lunch or evening meal using typical foods from that country. People could be encouraged to adopt a particular dress style pertaining to the chosen theme; appropriate music could be played as well. This idea could work particularly well if any of the residents are from a particular country because it could be viewed as a celebration of their culture.

Case study: Patricia

Patricia, one of the support workers in a day care facility, had recently received the *Hummingbird Bakery Cookbook* (Malouf 2009) as a birthday present. She thought it would be a good idea to try out some of the recipes such as the cupcakes with the older people attending the day centre. Patricia decided to ask another member of staff to assist her; she then asked some of the older people if they would be interested in such a group. Some of the male residents said they were interested in a baking group but not in baking cakes. Patricia then decided to run two groups – one for those interested in baking cupcakes and one for the male residents.

Discussion points:

- What type of baking activities might be more appropriate for males?

- With the baking of cupcakes, how might you tailor the activity to meet the needs of group members with varying abilities?

Case study: Linda

Linda used to be a professional baker. The manager of the day centre always ensured that people's birthdays were celebrated and used to arrange for a cake to be made by the chef. The day centre manager had the idea of encouraging Linda to work alongside the chef to make and decorate the cakes for people's birthdays.

If there is an opportunity for older people to work alongside you – for example, helping to lay the dining tables – consider what you are asking them to do and whether it is safe for them to do it. You may need to adapt the activity on the spot according to people's strengths and weaknesses – for example, asking them to lay just one table and placing the crockery on the table for them to sort out.

Other domestic activities can include tasks such as laundry if the setting permits – for example, within a care home. Older people could be encouraged to access the laundry room to go through the process of sorting their clothes, hand-washing small items or delicate clothing and perhaps using the washing machine for other items. People could also be encouraged to hang out their clothing – indoors or outdoors if facilities and the weather permits. Once clothing is dry, the process of sorting out clothing, folding and ironing, and putting it away completes the cycle.

Case study: Joan

Joan, one of the residents, liked to keep her room neat and tidy. She asked if she could have a Hoover® to clean her room and the care staff arranged for her to have access to the Hoover® on a regular basis. Joan was also given access to the small laundry trolley and once a week she would work with one of the care staff to sort out her laundry and take it down to the laundry room for washing, drying, ironing, folding and putting away.

Case study: Richard

Richard, the activity co-ordinator, wanted to start up a gardening group because a few of the older people had indicated an interest in renovating a neglected courtyard area within the grounds of the day centre facility. One day, Richard noticed that wooden pallets were used when supplies of food were being delivered to the day care facility, and he asked if some of them could be donated to the gardening group. The maintenance man broke up the pallets, made good the spare bits of wood and worked with a small group of older people who helped him to fit the pieces of wood together and then sand, varnish and paint them to make planters. Over a period of a few months, the courtyard area was completely transformed. The older people celebrated with an informal drinks party and invited the local mayor to unveil the new area.

Evaluation

Asking older people questions concerning their thoughts and feelings about participating in activities that come under life skills and interests will help facilitators to gauge whether they have been successful or not. This can be done on either a one-to-one or a group basis.

Exercise

Use the case study of Betty from Chapter 1. A wide range of life skills activities would potentially be suitable for Betty to encourage her to maintain independence with daily living activities. Which life skills activities do you think would be most suitable for Betty and why?

How to get started with life skills and interests groups

Task 1: Spring planting

What does the task involve?

Potting up wooden planters to use outdoors to grow plants.

What is needed?

Suitable containers for outdoor use, paint, paint brushes, compost and bulbs.

Instructions

Paint the planter, fill it with compost and plant some bulbs.

What could you do next?

Once the spring bulbs have faded, you could plant some runner beans, tomatoes or other suitable vegetables. One of the residents could take responsibility for looking after the planter and harvesting the vegetables, which the chef could then include in menus.

Task 2: 'Girls' night in'

What does the task involve?

Consult residents about having a designated 'girls' night in', the aim being to have a few hours one evening for each resident to have a pampering and makeover session.

What is needed?

Range of drinks, beauty box consisting of make-up, manicure implements, hairdressing implements.

Instructions

Create a relaxed atmosphere by serving some drinks and nibbles and playing some jazz-type music in the background. Get the residents to think about beauty regimes – you could offer face masks, hand manicures and nail polishing, make-up application, trying out different hairstyles and looking at clothing. The facilitator could consider if the more able residents are able to assist others with aspects of beauty care such as applying nail polish, brushing hair and so on.

What could you do next?

You could have a 'men's night in'. Think about what the content of this could be – for example, temporarily transforming the dining area into a pub-style room, setting up a bar and having activities available such as darts, snooker and cards.

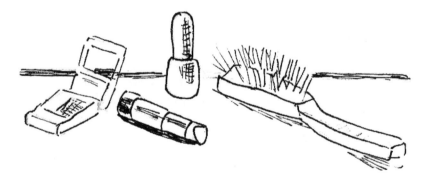

How to Facilitate Cognitive Activities for Stimulation with Groups and Individuals

What are cognitive based activities?

Cognition involves attention, concentration, decision making and problem solving. It covers a range of activities ranging from reading and discussion to puzzles, games and using computers. The activities can be a source of stimulation and enjoyment when older people are working together to solve puzzles, or sharing ideas as in creative writing. They can also be empowering, allowing people's opinions to be heard and enabling people to make decisions. Recently Cognitive Simulation Therapy (CST) has become a popular approach and was recommended by the National Institute for Health and Clinical Excellence (NICE) (2006) for people with mild to moderate dementia. CST involves themed group activity sessions in which tasks are aimed at strengthening cognitive capacity.

Selected literature in brief

Hurtley and Wenborn (2000) consider that cognitive based activities can:

- enhance the use of reasoning skills
- offer an opportunity for older people to make choices and decisions
- promote interaction

- provide a sense of competition

- enhance orientation

- promote lifelong learning for older people.

Spector *et al.* (2003) evaluated the effects of CST groups on cognition and quality of life for people with dementia in a single blind multi-centre randomised controlled trial. They found that CST groups appeared to improve both cognitive ability and quality of life for people with dementia. They also noted that participants liked the groups, which can be facilitated in a variety of settings – for example, indoor and outdoor gardening. In order to maintain the benefits, the authors contended that CST would need to be conducted on a regular long-term basis. One of the changes could be due to the learning environment during sessions that was designed to be appropriate for people with dementia. The focus of the sessions was on memory and integration of reminiscence and multisensory stimulation throughout the sessions. Stimulation in the group could improve cognition and might make participants feel more able to communicate.

Benham (2007) used innovative board games specially developed for older people with dementia attending a day hospital. According to her observations, board games offered structure and focus, creativity and imagination. They also generated communication and laughter, and enhanced life experiences of older people with dementia.

From the older person's perspective

The ability to participate in meaningful cognitive based activities can have an impact upon the well-being of older people and give them a sense of achievement. Cognitive based activities can be solitary, such as reading a magazine, or done in groups, such as Scrabble, but they are an essential component of lifelong learning and can help to maintain older people's orientation by presenting them with new challenges and tasks to accomplish, such as writing a poem.

From the facilitator's perspective

Engaging in a cognitive based activity can be a helpful talking point or a way of sharing information with an older person. In this way a facilitator can find out more about older people, their abilities, interests, strengths and areas that might pose difficulty. It may be that an older person has a particular talent – for example, for answering quizzes or developing strategies for board games such as chess. It may become apparent that some older people have skills that could be used further – as a bingo caller, for example.

The cognitive activities chart will help to identify suitable activities.

Cognitive activities chart

Beetle drives	Discussions	Puzzles
Bingo	Dominoes	Quizzes
Books	Draughts	Radio listening
Bridge	Hangman	Scrabble
Cards	Internet surfing	Sudoko
Chess	Jigsaws	Television viewing
Cinema club or film	Magazines	Word games
appreciation	Mastermind	Workbooks
Cluedo	Newspapers	
Computer games	Poetry reading	
Creative writing		
Crosswords		

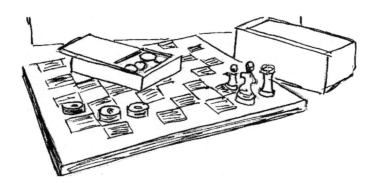

Planning

Assessment

One of the essential steps in the process requires a careful assessment of the older person's cognitive needs. This involves the following.

- Identifying the older person's interests, cognitive abilities and needs from some of the assessments such as the 'Client Profile Sheet' (Bender, Norris and Bauckman 1991), 'Reality Orientation Assessment' (Rimmer 1982), 'Simon's Nursing Assessment Manual' (O'Donovan 1996) and 'Personal History Profile' (Pool 2008).

- Matching the finding of assessments with the needs of the older person and aims of the individual or group work. Older people who are at 'planned' or 'exploratory' activity levels (Pool 2008) are likely to benefit from cognitive based activities. Although an older person at the 'planned' level is able to complete the activity, support may be needed in solving problems. Older people who are performing between levels 3 and 5 (Rimmer 1982) will also benefit from cognitive based group activities that have a focus on reality orientation.

Case study: Gerald

At a residents' meeting, activity worker Jonathan discussed a possible programme of events and activities. Gerald pointed out that he would like to know how to email his teenage granddaughter in Australia. Other residents also expressed an interest in keeping up with new technology. Jonathan set up a small weekly group using a computer in one of the lounges. Together the residents learned how to use the computer and the internet. Gerald was delighted to find out how to download a photograph of himself from Jonathan's digital camera and then send it by email to his granddaughter. He was very taken with this new form of contact that he can have with his family rather than waiting a long time for letters.

Case study: Day centre beetle drive

Chatting to the older people over lunch one day, Janice, a day centre support worker, found out that they all had very happy memories of going to a beetle drive in their youth. Janice decided to organise a beetle drive in the run-up to Christmas. There was much hilarity and fun as people threw the dice and drew the shape of a beetle. Richard added a hat and boots to his beetle, much to the amusement of the people sitting around him. Everyone enjoyed tea and cake and the small prizes for everyone taking part were an added treat to take home at the end of the day.

Deciding the format

When planning a cognitive based session, it is important to consider the following.

Will it be on an individual or a group basis?

If it is on an individual basis, where is the best place to do that?

If it is to be in a group, where will the session take place? (In either case, a quiet room with tables and chairs is preferred.)

What are the aims of the session?

Which cognitive based activities should be used? (The cognitive activities chart can be used as a starting point.)

What materials and equipment are needed for the session?

Will they need to be adapted so that everyone can complete the task? Do the domino pieces or the words on the puzzles need to be larger?

How much briefing do the facilitators and helpers require in order to assist with the smooth working progress of the session?

Will some people need additional support during the session? How will this be sensitively provided?

Preparing the room

Ensure that the room is set up with enough tables, chairs and equipment, and that these are placed within easy reach of participants and with adequate space for facilitators to move around easily to help the older people in the session. An appropriate level of lighting and a fairly quiet environment are essential to enable the older people to attend and complete the task(s) with minimum interruption.

Preparing equipment

Making sure that the facilitator has everything that will be needed to run the session and for the older people to carry out the task is essential to its success and ultimately to the level of enjoyment and satisfaction felt by the older people participating. It is likely that some of the equipment may need to be adapted to ease manipulation of, for example, large pieces of Scrabble or playing cards.

Implementation

Decide on the process because it may take several forms. A useful starting point could be to tell the older people what the task is and to enquire as to their familiarity with the activity. If they are not familiar with the activity, it may be useful to demonstrate and adapt it depending on the levels of skill and ability of the older people.

When providing help, judgment should be used to assess the level of help needed. Some older people may experience difficulty in completing some or all parts of the task. It is important that an individual is supported or prompted but the task should not be taken over by the facilitator.

Create an enabling environment to minimise the potential pressures experienced by some older people who may feel they are slow and being left behind with the task. Unless the cognitive based activities are ongoing, it is important that the task is completed within the time limits of the session so that everyone can gain a sense of achievement. Many cognitive based activities can be done in pairs or in teams.

Evaluation

Wenborn (2003) pointed out that some older people may feel that they have not performed as well as they used to. She suggested identifying the aspects of the cognitive based activities that have been valued and then using them again in subsequent sessions.

The following evaluation may serve the needs of both the older people and the facilitator for cognitive based groups. Notes should be made about the older people's engagement – in particular their ability to follow and complete the task(s) at hand or their ability to retain and acquire new learning (O'Donovan 1996).

Assessment of level of engagement by facilitator

Name of individual:
Name of facilitator:
Procedure: use the numbers 1–10 to rate the older person's performance
Social interaction   A little 1 2 3 4 5 6 7 8 9 10 A lot
Attention   A little 1 2 3 4 5 6 7 8 9 10 A lot
Engagement   A little 1 2 3 4 5 6 7 8 9 10 A lot
Cooperation   A little 1 2 3 4 5 6 7 8 9 10 A lot

Assessment of level of engagement by individual older person

Name of individual:
Name of facilitator:
Procedure: ask the older person to use the numbers 1–10 to rate self-perception of performance
Social interaction   A little 1 2 3 4 5 6 7 8 9 10 A lot
Attention   A little 1 2 3 4 5 6 7 8 9 10 A lot
Engagement   A little 1 2 3 4 5 6 7 8 9 10 A lot
Cooperation   A little 1 2 3 4 5 6 7 8 9 10 A lot

Ask the older person for ideas for future sessions.

Case study: Betty

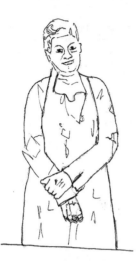

Having read her history, one of the activity co-ordinators asked if Betty would be interested in doing creative writing. This prompted Betty to reminisce about the past when she used to encourage her school pupils to get them to write 'poetry'. She was pleased when she was able to finish a piece of creative writing. This is Betty's poem.

'Weather Rhyme'

Zodiac zones in heavens dome
Constellations roaming
Struggle and strife
Stratosphere and atmosphere

Aquarius with her pitcher flowing
Snowflakes descending
The Albatross ascending
Apollo's extending light

The Mistral from a distant place
Icy and cold
Unrelenting blows
Down the valley face

Hush, the South trade stirs
Sahara's breezes rush and warm the snows
Velvet greens and silver streams
The crescent moon reflects in blue lagoons

Birds flocking, suddenly take flight
The cockerel's perch, lofty and bright
Spinning in vane
Oh! The weather it's as fickle as a feather.

Exercise: Betty's poem

How could you use Betty's poem to engage with her and empower her to tell you more? Do you work with an individual or group who would enjoy creative writing? Plan a session thinking about how you could inspire people to think creatively and write down their thoughts.

How to get started with cognitive based activities

Task 1: Newspapers

What does the task involve?

Getting together to use specific sections of newspapers or magazines for lifelong learning.

What is needed?

A few copies of the same issues of the newspapers or magazines.

Instructions

Buy papers and magazines that contain features and articles of general interest to the group. These could include, for example:

- local and national news
- current and old photographs of famous individuals or local dignitaries
- letters to the editor
- tips on healthcare
- crosswords.

In addition to reading and completing some of the activities such as crosswords, consider the following innovative ways of using newspapers and magazines:

Quiz time: encourage the older people to focus on particular pages or themes in the papers or magazines. Stage a quiz on the week's events. Individuals could work on their own, in pairs or in teams.

Viewpoint: consider how the paper has covered an important local issue. Find a news story that also carries an editorial comment. Compare the two styles of writing. Does the paper express an opinion in the news article? How do we distinguish between matters of fact and matters of opinion?

Letters to the Editor: study this page. What sorts of issue do people write letters about?

Crime: note the number and kinds of crimes reported in the newspaper. Which areas seem to have the highest number of crimes? What are the reasons for a high level of crime in a particular area? Has the area been famous for a high level of crime?

Word search: give everyone one sheet from a newspaper or magazine along with a pencil and paper. Ask them to begin at the top of the left-hand column of the newsprint and write down the first word discovered beginning with the letter A. Next they find a word beginning with the letter B, etc. When all the alphabet letters are found, ask them to write a sentence using the words written down in any order. If appropriate, invite everyone to read out their sentence – the one who has used the most words is voted to have written the most apt sentence and can be declared the winner (Dynes 1990).

What could you do next?

You could listen to or watch TV or radio programmes, raise and discuss relevant issues or write to the local newspaper about issues raised in the newspapers.

Task 2: Debates

What does the task involve?

This is a group activity for older people who get together to debate topical issues. Debating can give older people practice in speaking and having their opinions heard. It also makes them more aware of issues that surround day-to-day life and gives them the different points of view that come with every issue.

What is needed?

A range of topical debates.

Instructions

Appoint a Chair and have an equal number of proponents and opponents and an audience. Take it in turns for each side to put forward their arguments and points of view. Allocate a specific time limit for each debater.

The following are possible topics that could be debated:

- Single-sex schools provide the best method of education.
- Current screen culture damages the behaviour of children.
- Babies don't suffer when mothers return to work.
- Overeating pregnant mothers raise the obesity risk for their babies.

To conclude the session, the Chair will summarise the key points and ask for a vote from the audience.

What could you do next?

The group could get their views published in their local newsletter.

Task 3: Giving a minute talk

What does the task involve?

This is a group activity for individuals who enjoy giving brief talks on any topic.

What is needed?

A range of topics.

Instructions

Appoint a Chair and invite some older people to form teams. There should also be an audience. Invite an older person to give a talk for one minute without a single hesitation, repetition or deviation about any given topic, such as a washing machine. Hosted like the 'Just a Minute' programme on the radio, the Chair will pick one of the following topics in a random manner:

- Aeroplanes.
- Batteries.
- Clouds.
- Computers.
- Donkeys.
- Fur.
- Pigeons.
- The Queen.
- Submarines.
- Typewriters.

If the older people manage to talk continuously, they will score a point for their team. If they repeat themselves or deviate from the topic, they will not gain a point. At the end, the team who has the most points wins.

What could you do next?

You could arrange an intergenerational talking group.

Task 4: Lifelong learning group

What does the task involve?

This is a group for individuals who decide to use their spare time to become adult learners.

What is needed?

A group of individuals with an interest in lifelong learning, and a facilitator, chairs, tables, flipcharts and pens.

Instructions

On a flipchart, write the skills each older person has and the skills the person would like to have. Look at the list of topics and identify the one that most group members would like to learn, such as how to undertake internet shopping. Get the group member to thought shower the different steps needed to be done and the deadline to achieve their goal of internet shopping, for example.

Step 1 Gain access to a computer.

Step 2 Go to a relevant shopping website.

Step 3 Click on the items you wish to purchase.

Step 4 Proceed to the checkout.

Step 5 Complete the relevant details to pay for the items purchased.

Step 6 Make a note of your order details and purchase code.

Step 7 Await delivery

Step 8 Unpack the goods and check against order!

What could you do next?

You could contact Learndirect, which provides information and advice about learning and leisure; Age UK, which has produced online and downloadable guides on making the most of the internet; BBC WebWise Basics which are courses for people who don't know how to use a keyboard, mouse or computer screen; and Pass IT On, which is an online course to teach basic and advanced computing skills.

CHAPTER 13

How to Facilitate a Carer Support Group

What is a carer support group?

Carer support can take on many meanings, from help with emotional problems and practical information to assistance with coping strategies. Such groups consider people's needs and what is appropriate to support them in their caring role. For many people caring is a journey where their needs and situation can change with time, especially if they are looking after someone with a progressive degenerative condition. Carers may be supporting people to live at home or supporting people living in formal care situations; they may find their caring role evolves from the first to the second situation. They can also be of many ages: the partners, children or other relatives of the cared-for. Carers UK estimate that there are 6 million carers of all ages in the UK. Nationally, with the rising number of older people in the population, it is significant that older people are not only being cared for but are also the providers of care for an older partner. The caring experience can have lasting effects upon the person long after the cared-for has died. It may be that, when their caring role ends, carers may still have needs that can be met by attending a family carer support group although they are technically no longer carers. Carers can play an important peer group supporting role by helping new carers, listening to their stories and, in doing so, showing that there is life after caring.

Selected literature in brief

Heathcote, Newton and Chia (2007) studied carers of people with dementia attending a regular musical reminiscence session where for part of the session the cared-for worked with volunteers, allowing carers time to talk to each other. They found that family carers valued this opportunity to meet people in a similar situation, to talk and to make new friends. Carers stressed the importance of companionship, the 'safe' environment and the feelings of hope and of not being alone that the group provided.

Mitchell (1996) compared six carer support groups in Scotland and examined the impact of organisational structure, defined as their link to service providers, and the client group focus. It was found that both influenced the character and operation of the group. Mitchell stressed the similarity in care needs for emotional support and information but also highlighted the systematic differences in the emphasis of groups, concluding that a variety of care support groups are required to meet these differing needs.

Charlesworth *et al.* (2009) evaluated a 'Positive Caring Programme' provided by the Alzheimer's Society for carers. This was a small sample where the carers were predominantly women aged between 43 and 81. Carers showed higher scores for knowledge and coping and lower scores for level of anxiety following the carer support sessions.

From the carer's perspective

Heathcote and Chia (2009) suggest that the caring role can deny people access to social situations and activity. Many carers feel very alone in their caring role, coping with physical caring and financial and legal situations, often with nobody to talk to and discuss matters with. If they are older people themselves, they may need support for their own physical conditions, and yet the primary focus is often on the people they care for before their own needs as carers are considered. Attending a carer support group can help provide support for carers in many ways. Being able to talk to other carers and facilitators who understand their situation and what they are going through, to share information and the chance to 'let off steam' that support groups provide can be very valuable to carers.

Case study: Frances

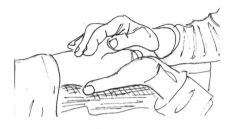

Frances is 82 years old and cares at home for her husband who is 85 and has dementia. After a particularly stressful and sleepless week looking after her husband, Frances arrived at the support group looking anxious. As soon as she sat down, she started to cry. She seemed to gain some comfort from the other carers in the group who identified with her concerns and fears. Frances held the facilitator's hand throughout the session and at the end commented that she had been helped because she had been able to show her emotions, something that she could not do at home.

From the facilitator's perspective

Support groups for carers can make a significant difference to the lives of some carers and facilitators can feel that they have played a part in helping people at a difficult stage of their lives. By providing this support and maintaining people in their own homes, carer support groups can also reduce the need for hospitalisation and long-term care for the cared-for.

However, working at this level and listening to the difficult emotional situations faced by carers, some of which may be outside the facilitator's control, can be stressful for facilitators. Facilitators may also need support and ongoing training to carry out their role effectively.

Planning

What type of carer support group?

Two possible models for carer support groups are:

1. A group that carers attend on their own while care is provided for the cared-for at home. This structure gives carers a break from caring and a chance to do something on their own. This type of group may require facilitators to organise care for the

person at home that is acceptable to the carer, and transport for the carer to attend the group sessions.

2. A group where carers and their cared-for attend together with a carer support element during the session. A structure where both attend may be less stressful because when carers know that the cared-for is there, they feel less anxious. This type of group will require facilitators arranging for people to look after and work with the cared-for onsite in a different room – for example, while carers have their own separate time to attend the support group – and for transport for both to reach and leave the venue. Such a model effectively involves organising two groups and this may cut across lunch time and involve additional catering.

Where to find the carers?

When setting up a new group or finding members for an established group, carers may come by referral from doctors and other healthcare professionals or from contact with local charitable organisations helping older people, such as the Alzheimer's Society and Age UK (formerly Age Concern and Help the Aged). Local advertisements in surgeries, hospitals and newspapers may also find new carers. Some carers may also wish to join a group because they have heard about it from other people.

Funding

Considering the following may help you in seeking funding for a carer support group.

Do you need to find funding by applying for grants to run the group?

Will a local company sponsor your support group?

Do you intend to charge carers for part of the session, such as making a donation towards tea or coffee, lunch and outings?

Working in partnership with other groups may help facilitators to find funding. Some partners may be able to provide help 'in kind', such as providing a room for the group to meet free of charge, or providing volunteers to help with making tea and coffee.

More information about initiating groups is available in Chapter 6.

Finding a venue

The following points should be considered when choosing a venue for the support group that is within budget.

Is the venue easy to reach by all forms of transport including public transport?

Is there parking space, including for minibus transport?

Does the venue provide the space required, separate rooms for carers and cared-for, small meeting rooms for one-to-one advice?

Is the atmosphere, temperature, lighting, seating and general ambience suitable?

Does the venue provide a relaxed setting for people to meet?

How much room preparation (and room restoring) will be involved, such as moving chairs and tables?

Are there good disabled access facilities?

Are there good toilet facilities?

Is there a kitchen to make refreshments?

How long will you need to use the venue for each session?

Planning a programme

Facilitators also need to consider the needs of the carers and how to support them so that everyone receives the attention and information they need. One way may be to ask carers what they hope to gain from attending the sessions.

Dröes *et al.* (2009) described a Dutch carer support group where the programme changed weekly using the following elements.

- Discussion groups to provide emotional support.

- Informative meetings to provide factual information, usually provided by specialists.

- A counselling hour, which cared-for and carers shared.

- Joint activities for the carer and cared-for, to provide recreation and to expand their social network.

Chambers, Ryan and Connors (2001) found that the majority of carers in their study had a constant need for support and information, and to find a balance between the physical and emotional demands of caring. Supporting carers with the knowledge they need could include organising a programme of specialist speakers on such topics as medical issues surrounding conditions and treatment, diet and eating issues, legal issues including power of attorney and financial issues such as benefit entitlement. Practical advice such as moving and handling may also be appropriate for some carers. However, it is also important that topic areas are not too 'information heavy': having time to laugh and be recharged for a short time can be very beneficial for carers. Priority should be given to relaxation and 'time out' for carers by the provision of relaxation sessions, 'pampering', exercise, aromatherapy and hand massage.

Coping strategies for carers

Chambers *et al.* (2001) found that carers on their own were learning how to deal with their situation by trial and error and that there was a general feeling of abandonment. Carers commented that lack of knowledge was stressful and that with accurate information it was easier to put coping strategies in place. This study showed that carers coped in different ways and that their strategies reflected personal, environmental and cultural factors. General acceptance, taking practical action and simple measures were suggested by carers to help them cope. These included going into the garden, walking into another room for a while, trying to relax over a cup of tea and thinking positive thoughts. Many mentioned the importance of being allowed to let off steam.

Given these points, it would seem that support groups should address coping strategies that could be used in different situations in order to improve carer competence and well-being. Chambers *et al.* (2001) urged the facilitators of carer support groups to be 'proactive in assessing and meeting carers' emotional and support needs'.

Exercise: Planning a programme

Think about how, as a facilitator, you could provide helpful information for the people in your group. Make a list of the things you would need to consider. You could start with: Who will be attending the group? What type of information will they need? This list could then help you to focus on planning a programme for the group, how you will arrange the group, and the type of information and leaflets you will need to provide in sessions.

Implementation

Structure for the carer support session

Implementing a clear structure that is followed each week, such as having refreshments on arrival, a beginning and end to the session, and the opportunity for carers to spend time talking to each other can help the session run smoothly.

Case study: Support group for carers of people with dementia

Carers arrived at different times according to transportation and were greeted by the facilitators. Their cared-for were at home with substitute carers. Over tea, coffee and biscuits, some carers chatted to each other, others immediately went to facilitators to discuss issues of concern. When everyone had arrived, the main facilitator welcomed the group members, who were sitting informally in a horseshoe shape. The first part of the session was a talk from a guest speaker during which there were questions and the chance for carers to share information. One man particularly mentioned how much he valued having someone else to talk to and how difficult he found caring for his wife who had limited conversation due to her memory loss. The end of the session consisted of providing information and addressing particular issues that were affecting people. Carers then talked to each other again and left at different times, the whole session lasting about two and a half hours.

Communication between carers

Allowing carers time to talk to each other and share experiences is vital to a successful carer support group, and time should be given for refreshments, sharing and listening to each other.

Maintaining support

Providing and updating information about resources and services is also important. Some carer support groups are restrained by budgets and can only offer a service for a limited period of time. If this is the case, it is important that carers continue to feel supported and this may be by the facilitator suggesting other groups they could attend. After attending a support group, some carers may feel empowered to continue to meet informally without a facilitator, such as getting together for lunch.

Ownership of the carer support group

It may be applicable to allow the carers attending the group some ownership of the programme and choice of talks and speakers. Some carer support groups also organise extra activities for group members, such as outings and lunches for carers and their cared-for.

Evaluation

As the needs of carers are ongoing and constantly changing, it is important to review regularly the group and the level of support provided. It may be applicable to ask carers what they hope to gain from the sessions before they attend, then to ask for their feelings once they have started attending and to repeat the evaluation throughout their time at the carer support group. In this way, changing needs can be identified.

Heathcote et al. (2007) evaluated a group for people with dementia and their carers by using questionnaires at the start of the sessions, and then again several months later. This was a small sample of eight couples. Prior to attending the group, feelings of apprehension were expressed: 'apprehensive because we can't mix or go out a lot' and 'afraid he will disrupt things, be too demanding and we will not be able to attend again', for example. With the second set of questionnaires, carers reported more positive responses: people said the group offered them 'companionship', 'fun', a 'change of scenery' and 'the chance to relax knowing that my husband is enjoying his day out and that I am not totally responsible'.

The reactions of facilitators towards the group and individual needs should also be evaluated. This could be done by having discussion and feedback at the end when carers have left. Confidentiality is a key issue. One facilitator may have noticed a concern that others have not seen. Sometimes carers choose one facilitator to 'unburden themselves' to. While those issues should be treated confidentially, they may inform a future approach and the type of help required, and they should not be ignored. Deciding how and when it is appropriate to deal with this information is an important part of the evaluation process. The effect on the facilitator of supporting people should also be considered. Debriefing time could also include facilitators discussing how listening to other people's situations is affecting them both inside and outside their facilitating role, with emphasis placed on coping strategies for facilitators. For more information on ways to evaluate, see Chapter 14.

Case study: Supporting Sam

Sam is an only child and has been very worried about his mother, Betty, for some time. He has found it increasingly difficult supporting her to live independently while also working full time (for Betty's full case study and profile see Chapters 1 and 2). When Betty was recently admitted to hospital, diagnosed with Alzheimer's and prescribed Aricept, Sam felt bewildered and shocked.

He had thought his mother was just depressed. Sam feels quite alone in dealing with his mother's diagnosis and medication: he does not know how to deal with a condition he does not understand, and he is fearful about what the future will bring.

Exercise

How would you help Sam? What type of carer support do you feel would be most appropriate?

CHAPTER 14

The Importance of Evaluating Work with Older People

What is evaluation?

Evaluation is a crucial part of any intervention: without evaluation, it is not possible to state critically that the outcome of an intervention has been successful. Intervention in the context of this book can be construed as group or individual work with an older person. Evaluation is defined as:

> ...a component of a broader assessment process. It involves the collection of data to enable the therapist to make a judgement about the amount of a specific construct of interest (such as degree of range of movement or level of independence in an activity of daily living) or to make a judgement about the value of an intervention for delivering the desired outcome for a person or the value of a service for delivering outcomes of relevance to the client population. Evaluation often involves data being collected at two time points in order to measure effect and also can involve the translation of observations to numerical scores. (Laver Fawcett 2007, p.6)

Outcome measures form a part of the broader evaluation process with a narrow focus on establishing whether an intervention has been effective. Standardisation has already been discussed in Chapter 4 on assessments. Within the context of outcome measures, an example of a standardised instrument is the Canadian Occupational Performance Measure (Law *et al.* 2005).

The benefits of evaluation include opportunities to:

- review the purpose of the intervention

- justify the use of resources (time, staffing, materials, room required, etc.)

- justify the intervention being repeated

- justify the need for any changes required

- identify the need for a different approach

- identify the need for more training for facilitators

- self-monitor performance when facilitating groups and working with people on an individual basis.

After a session has been concluded, the facilitators involved need to review actual performance and achievements against the original session plan. This evaluation takes two forms:

1. Evaluation of each group member's performance. This need not be particularly detailed, but it does need to be sensitive enough to monitor change and progress.

2. Evaluation of the performance of the facilitator in meeting the learning objectives.

Methods of evaluation

There are various frameworks and tools that can be employed to conduct an evaluation – whether with facilitators, older people, or indeed, as self-evaluation. Some of the frameworks and tools are formal in that they are published and widely recognised; others are done in a more informal way. It is important to consider for what purpose you need to evaluate and who is interested in the outcomes – for example, managers, key stakeholders, other staff or facilitators, older people or relatives of older people?

For a more informal means of evaluation, whether with clients or facilitators, consider the various means by which you can achieve this:

- Verbal feedback – collect ideas onto a flipchart or sheet of paper.

- Jot down words or short phrases on Post-it® notes.

- Video evaluation.

- Questionnaire.

- Use of photographs.

- Use of observation sheets and tools such as those recommended by Sheard (2008).

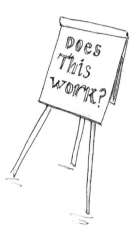

Bender, Norris and Bauckham (1991) recommend that evaluation takes place as soon as possible after a group has finished because this aids recall of what went on during the group.

Plan, Do, Study, Act

The NHS Institute for Innovation and Improvement is centred on 'support[ing] the NHS to transform healthcare for patients and the public by rapidly developing and spreading new ways of working, new technology and world class leadership'. As part of this vision, there is an emphasis on quality and value – that is, providing advice on improving the quality and value of care. One such model advocated is the 'model for improvement', which focuses on key questions leading to a process cycle with four distinct stages to work through – Plan, Do, Study, Act (PDSA).

The NHS Institute for Innovation and Improvement explains the four different stages of the PDSA cycle as follows:

Plan – the change to be tested or implemented.

Do – carry out the test or change.

Study – data before and after the change and reflect on what was learned.

Act – plan the next change cycle or full implementation.

Using the PDSA cycle enables changes to be tested on a small scale before being implemented more widely. An example of how this cycle might be used in the context of working with older people in group settings is as follows.

Plan

This part of the cycle is broken down into three steps to ensure a thorough understanding of what it is you plan to change.

Your aim

To produce a new activities programme within the local centre where you work. Following a recent inspection by the National Care Standards Commission, the recommendations included the need to review the existing activities programme because of poor attendance by older people.

ORIGINAL PROCESS

Repetition of current activities programme for several years.

Some of the activities are inappropriate (e.g. use of activities aimed at a young age group [children]).

Demotivated older people and reduced quality of life.

Demotivated facilitators.

Poor inspection result.

New process

Implementation of new activities programme.

Motivated older people and facilitators.

Increased attendance at activities.

Better use of resources.

Improved re-inspection result.

Objectives (What changes can you make? What do you need to do?)

- Review current activities programme. How is it organised? Are there any written records pertaining to the activity programme? Is there a nominated person who takes responsibility for activities? Are facilitators trained to prepare, implement and evaluate activities? Is the current programme relevant and appropriate for the older people attending the centre?

- Consult with older people. Working in partnership with older people is important because you need to seek their views. In doing so, they may be more likely to participate in the activities planned. Consult with older people and residents on what activity programme they would prefer within the centre; capture these onto flipchart paper.

- Design flyer. Advertising a new activities programme is important so that both facilitators and older people are aware of the changes. Consider how you will design the flyer to attract attention. You also need to consider the format in which you produce this. What about people with visual or cognitive impairments? Will they be able to see and understand the contents of the flyer?

- Draw up activity plan and circulate to facilitators and older people for comment and feedback.

- Identify resources and agree start date. What resources are required to implement the new activities programme? Think about facilitator availability, rooms required, materials, costs involved.

Measurement

Increased attendance by older people at activities planned and implemented by the centre to 75 per cent by the end of six weeks.

Do

Implement the new activities programme within the centre for six weeks and increase attendance by 75 per cent. Review the current activities programme; because of the repetition of the current activities programme without a review, some activities are inappropriate, demotivating older people and facilitators. Attendance on the current activities programme is virtually negligible.

Study

This part of the cycle looks at whether the change (i.e. the new activities programme) has had the desired effect. Are there any issues? Did it work? Are any changes needed to the programme? What is the attendance rate of older people at each activity?

Act

The final part of the cycle concerns the full implementation of the new activities programme or the need to try out the programme again with further changes.

It is likely that you will need to repeat the PDSA cycle several times in order to demonstrate an improvement.

Older people's evaluation

Seeking the views of an older person you have been working with is important because they are on the receiving end. Conducting an evaluation is also an important means of empowering older people, involving them in possible decision making with regard to changing aspects of the intervention the next time it is implemented. Possible prompts include:

> Did you enjoy the activity?

> Did you understand the reason for the activity?

Did you feel able to take part fully in the activity?

Was the facilitator able to communicate clearly what you had to do?

If you experienced any difficulties, were you given help to overcome these?

What changes, if any, are needed next time?

Would you attend this type of activity again?

Refer to the section earlier in this chapter on the different methods of evaluation because it is important to consider that some older people may not feel comfortable vocalising their thoughts about a group.

Group evaluation

Any method of evaluation should include questions. Ultimately, evaluation is as useful as facilitators allow it to be. If it is carried out without any reference back to the running of the session, then it is ineffective; if it leads to better training opportunities for older people and helps facilitators to refine and develop their leadership skills, then it is useful.

The following questions serve as useful prompts for monitoring the effectiveness of the activities engaged in with older people.

How successful was the activity?

Were the session aims and objectives achieved?

Were there any problems? If so, how did you manage them?

Could you have managed these problems differently?

What was the outcome of the activity? Did people enjoy it or not?

Which parts of the activity were successful and not successful?

Did anything go wrong?

What, if anything, would improve the activity?

Do you need to alter the activity in any way before you repeat it?

Staff or self-evaluation

On a more personal level, it may be useful to ask someone such as a manager, supervisor or mentor to observe your performance in facilitating a group and to provide objective feedback to help evaluate performance. Consideration needs to be given as to what aspect of your performance you want the observer to focus on.

Possible prompt questions for the observer include the following.

Were the session plan and aims clear and comprehensive?

Was the environment appropriate?

Was the room adequately prepared and set up?

Did the facilitator clearly state the aims of the session?

Was the facilitator clear and easy to understand when facilitating the group?

Did the facilitator respond appropriately to any unforeseen events?

Did the facilitator utilise appropriate non-verbal body language?

Did the group have a sense of structure (e.g. introduction, warm up, main activity, cooling down, conclusion)?

Reflective practice

Reflective practice is a process of self-monitoring and charting one's personal and professional development. Within the healthcare professions – for example, occupational therapy and physiotherapy – the requirement by the relevant professional bodies (College of Occupational Therapists and the Chartered Society of Physiotherapy) and the regulatory body, the Health Professions Council, places a requirement upon the therapist to maintain a continuing professional development (CPD) portfolio. This ensures that the therapist retains state registration as a healthcare professional. Non-professionals such as staff or facilitators who work with older people may also benefit from engaging in reflective practice and maintaining a CPD portfolio.

Case study: Michael

Michael, a care worker, has monthly supervision with the manager of the care home where he works. He finds this a useful process to ensure that he is meeting the aims of his current role. He also has an opportunity to discuss whether there are any problems arising and what can be done to help resolve these. The manager has decided to promote Michael into the role of activities co-ordinator and has suggested that he start to formalise his learning using a range of reflective tools. Michael is in agreement with this because he eventually wants to train to be a healthcare professional, and he feels that building up a professional profile will help consolidate his new role and subsequent skills, knowledge and attitudes acquired.

Reflective tools

A variety of reflective tools may be employed to monitor personal and professional development. These may include reflective diaries, critical incident logs, SWOB analyses and personal action plans. In using these, people build up profiles of their experience and capture the development of their skills, knowledge and attitudes gleaned from a range of situations or events encountered within the workplace or other relevant setting. The reflective tools can capture both positive and negative situations and events so, for example, a critical incident log does not necessarily have negative connotations: using this tool can be used to capture a positive learning experience. Reflective practice, therefore, is a form of self-evaluation. Stewart (2004) stresses that a portfolio can be used as a reflective and critical tool that facilitates professional development. Some organisations may have a process of supervision that provides an opportunity to talk through aspects of the job.

Within this section, some of the reflective tools that may prove useful are listed. Remember that more than one tool may be used in relation to one particular event because each tool offers a slightly different method of reflection. By using a variety of tools, it is possible to work your way thoroughly through a significant learning event by capturing different aspects and to achieve a sense of learning from this. Reflective practice should occur on a regular basis and will need to fit in with your work commitments. A few hours a month is a good idea. For a more comprehensive overview of reflective practice, refer to wider literature.

Exercise

Create a portfolio and divide this into different sections such as reflective diary, critical incidents, SWOB analyses and personal action plan.

REFLECTIVE DIARIES

The use of reflective diaries enables you to think about situations you have encountered and the thoughts, feelings and emotions experienced. You could think about including photographs of your work – for example, during and after activity sessions with residents or group members. You could also include quotes you have heard from the older people you work with regarding their perspectives on an activity you have done with them; this will enable you to evaluate the activity and to think about how you could do things differently or the same next time.

Exercise

Try starting a reflective diary; complete an entry every few days for the next two weeks. Figure 14.1 provides an example of a diary completed by a support worker in a day centre.

Date	Reflective diary
12.12.10	Today I ran a reminiscence group in the day care centre for older people where I was working for the first time. I was feeling nervous about it because I had been planning it for quite some time and my manager was going to be observing me as part of my college qualifications. Before the start of this activity I had given my manager a copy of my intended session plan so that he could see what my group aims were.
	The group was due to start at 11 a.m. At 10.50 a.m., I began to get people together and I got rather flustered as I realised I was not going to achieve a prompt 11 a.m. start. I couldn't really ask anyone else to help me because I had not told anyone about this group and they all had other tasks to attend to that day.
	Finally, at 11.10, everyone was in the activities room and I was ready to start. Because of time constraints, I missed out the introductory part of the session so this meant there was no 'warm up' to the activity. I just felt flustered the whole time and could not remember half of what I had intended to do because I had not prepared the materials as well as I thought I had in that I had borrowed a reminiscence box from the local library but had not gone through the contents. Also, I realised that I should have picked an overall theme to discuss with the group because it seemed to be lacking in structure. Despite all this, some of the people seemed to get some enjoyment out of the activity, but I need to find a way of formally evaluating this.
	I ran out of time because we had to finish by midday for lunch so this meant there was no winding down or conclusion to the group. I didn't think the group had gone that well and felt rather disappointed with my performance.
	My manager was encouraging though and for next supervision has asked me to think about what went well and why, what did not go so well and why, and what I would do differently next time.

Figure 14.1 Sample of reflective diary extract

CRITICAL INCIDENT LOGS

The writing up of critical incidents enables you to think in depth about a particular 'incident' – something that has happened that you feel is important for a particular reason, whether positive or negative. Consider the following questions.

What is the critical incident?

What did I learn?

How did I acquire the learning?

How have I applied this learning in my practice? (Cross 1997, p.42)

There are more questions that can be asked but for the purposes of this book, we have limited them to four.

Exercise

Using the questions outlined in this section, think about a particular incident, either positive or negative, that occurred recently. Now relate that incident and answer the questions using the critical incident template in Table 14.1.

Table 14.1: Critical incident template

What was the critical incident?	I was appointed key worker for one of the residents and was assisting the person in getting washed and dressed.
What did I learn?	The importance of taking time to listen to people and to get to know them. By doing this, I could build up a profile of their likes and dislikes. It meant that I was able to offer more personalised care (e.g. when assisting them getting up in the morning, I encouraged them to choose what clothes they wanted to wear and to become more independent with getting washed and dressed).
How did I acquire the learning?	Through observing more experienced key workers in action.
How have I applied this learning in my practice?	My key worker role has increased in that I now have five residents whom I am responsible for. I have applied the principle of listening and getting to know them and I am able to disseminate this knowledge to other care staff within the home.

SWOB ANALYSES

A SWOB analysis is a useful tool to encourage thinking about various aspects of a situation. It is useful to do this exercise either individually or within a group situation – for instance, during a staff meeting. An example might be in relation to reviewing the resources available in preparation for setting up a carer support group in the community.

Exercise

Using the SWOB template in Table 14.2, add to the strengths, weaknesses, opportunities and barriers in relation to a situation such as that just described.

Table 14.2: SWOB analysis

Strengths	Weaknesses
Local GP and representative from Age UK keen to get a carer support group up and running in the local community.	Current lack of staff who will commit to this project.
Opportunities	**Barriers**
To work alongside key stakeholders such as local GP and Age UK representative. Use of local village hall to host carer support meetings.	Local village hall not always available on a regular basis.

The next stage of this process is to think about how you can continue to work on the strengths, turn the weaknesses into strengths, exploit the opportunities and work around the barriers.

PERSONAL ACTION PLAN

Personal action plans are a good means of self-monitoring personal development. These could be shared with your line manager, supervisor or mentor. By compiling these action plans within a personal folder, it is possible to chart professional growth in terms of capturing skills, knowledge and attitudes.

Exercise

The example in Table 14.3 is of an exercise plan in relation to planning and implementing an exercise group. Can you think of another scenario that you could use in order to develop an action plan?

Table 14.3: Personal action plan

Objectives	Strategies	Resources	By when
These should adhere to the SMART principle and be specific, measurable, achievable, realistic and timed.	What strategies will you use to achieve your objective?	What resources do you need in order to achieve your objective?	By when will you have achieved your objective?
Example:	Example:	Example:	Example:
To plan and implement a one-hour exercise group, twice weekly, to run for a total of six weeks.	Liaise with manager. Design flyer to advertise group. Identify co-leader. Liaise with visiting physiotherapist. Shadow physiotherapist running an exercise group for older people at local hospital. Produce session plan for a one-hour exercise group with variations.	Book large sitting room. Purchase gym balls, cones, therabands. Visit medical library to search for relevant literature on running exercise groups.	Within one month of discussing this plan with line manager.

References

Introduction

College of Occupational Therapists and National Association for Providers of Activities for Older People (2007) *Activity Provision: Benchmarking Good Practice in Care Homes.* London: College of Occupational Therapists.

Finlay, L. (2000) 'When Actions Speak Louder: Groupwork in Occupational Therapy.' In O. Manor (ed.) *Ripples: Groupwork in Different Settings.* London: Whiting and Birch.

Chapter 1

Allen, J. (2008) *Older People and Well Being.* London: Institute for Public Policy Research.

Alzheimer's Society (2010a) *Understanding and Respecting the Person with Dementia.* London: Alzheimer's Society. Available at www.alzheimers.org.uk/factsheet/524, accessed on 13 December 2010.

Alzheimer's Society (2010b) 'My name is not dementia.' London: Alzheimer's Society. Available at http://alzheimers.org.uk/site/scripts/documents_info.php?documentID=1339, accessed on 30 April 2011.

Atkinson, K. (2004) 'SWOT Analysis: A Tool for CPD.' In S.H. Chia and D. Harrison (eds) *Tools for Continuing Professional Development.* Dinton: Quay Books.

Bowling, A., Gabriel, Z., Banister, D. and Sutton, S. (2003) 'Assessing quality of life in healthy older people.' *Journal of Nursing and Residential Care 5*, 11, 539–541.

Byers-Connon, S., Lohman, H.L. and Padilla, R.L. (2004) *Occupational Therapy with Elders.* St Louis, MO: Elsevier Mosby.

Davis, S. (ed.) (2006) *Rehabilitation – The Use of Theories and Models in Practice.* Edinburgh: Elsevier Churchill Livingstone.

Kitwood, T. (1997) *Dementia Reconsidered: The Person Comes First.* Buckingham: Open University Press.

Mountain, G. (2004) *Occupational Therapy with Older People.* London: Whurr.

National Institute for Health and Clinical Excellence (NICE) (2008) *Occupational Therapy Interventions and Physical Activity Interventions to Promote the Mental Well Being of Older People in Primary Care and Residential Care.* London: NICE.

Owen, T. (2006) *My Home Life Quality of Life in Care Homes*. London: Help the Aged.

Quality of Life Research Unit (2010) *Quality of Life*. Toronto, Ontario: University of Toronto. Available at www.utoronto.ca/qol, accessed on 13 December 2010.

Social Institute for Excellence (SCIE) (2010) *The Dignity in Care Campaign*. London: SCIE. Available at www.dignityincare.org.uk/DignityCareCampaign, accessed on 20 November 2010.

Stokes, G. and Goudie, F. (2003) *The Essential Dementia Care Handbook*. Bicester: Speechmark Publishing Ltd.

Victor, C.R., Scambler, S.J., Shah, S. and Cook, D. (2004) 'Are You Lonesome Tonight? The Social World of Older People.' Agenet Research Network Meeting. Reading: University of Reading.

Woodhouse, J. (2006) 'Person-centred care for older people in mental health.' *Therapy Weekly 16*, 7–9.

World Health Organization (WHO) (2010) *International Classification of Functioning, Disability and Health (ICF)*. Geneva: WHO. Available at www.who.int/classifications/icf/en, accessed on 13 December 2010.

Chapter 2

Bender, M., Norris, A. and Bauckham, P. (1994) *Groupwork with the Elderly*. Bicester: Winslow Press.

Brooker, D. (2001) 'Therapeutic Activity.' In C. Cantley (ed.) *A Handbook of Dementia Care*. Buckingham: Open University Press.

Care Quality Commission (2009) *The State of Health Care and Adult Social Care*. London: Care Quality Commission.

Cattan, M., White, M., Bond, J. and Learmouth, A. (2005) 'Preventing social isolation and loneliness among older people: A systematic review of health promotion interventions.' *Ageing and Society 25*, 1, 41–67.

Commission for Social Care Inspection (CCSI) (2006) *Social Care Should be Individual, not Institutional – More Money Needed but Improvements Should Begin Immediately*. London: CSCI. Cited in C. MacBrayne (2007) 'Therapeutic activities for older people.' *Journal of Nursing and Residential Care 9*, 11, 537–539.

Department of Health (2003) *Care Homes for Older People: National Minimum Standards and the Care Homes Regulations* (3rd edition, revised). London: Department of Health.

Finlay, L. (2000) 'When Actions Speak Louder: Groupwork in Occupational Therapy.' In O. Manor (ed.) *Ripples Groupwork in Different Settings.* London: Whiting and Birch.

Garvin, C.D., Gutierrez, L.M. and Galinsky, M.J. (2004) *Handbook of Social Work with Groups.* New York, NY: The Guilford Press.

Glass, T.A., Mendes de Leon, C., Marottoli, R.A. and Berkman, L.T. (1999) 'Population based study of social and productive activities as predictors of survival among elderly Americans.' *British Medical Journal 319,* 8, 478–483.

Heathcote, J. (2005) 'Choosing an individual reminiscence approach.' *Journal of Nursing and Residential Care 7,* 2, 78–80.

Leary, S. (1994) *Activities for Personal Growth.* Sydney: Maclennan & Petty.

MacBrayne, C. (2007) 'Therapeutic activities for older people.' *Journal of Nursing and Residential Care 9,* 11, 537–539.

Mold, F., Fitzpatrick, J.M. and Roberts, J.D. (2005) 'Caring for ethnic older people in nursing care homes.' *British Journal of Nursing 41,* 11, 601–606.

Mountain, G. (2004) *Occupational Therapy with Older People.* London: Whurr.

Mountain, G. and Moore, J. (1995) 'Quality of Life with Older People.' Unpublished study. Leeds: University of Leeds.

Owen, T. (2006) *My Home Life Quality of Life in Care Homes.* London: Help the Aged.

Peck, C. and Hong, C.S. (1994) *Living Skills for Mentally Handicapped People.* London: Croom Helm.

Perrin, T., May, H. and Anderson, E. (2010) *Well Being in Dementia.* Edinburgh: Churchill Livingstone Elsevier.

Tester, S., Hubbard, G., Downs, M., MacDonald, C. and Murphy, J. (2004) 'What does quality of life mean for frail residents?' *Journal of Nursing and Residential Care 6,* 2, 89–92.

Walsh, D. (1993) *Groupwork Activities.* Bicester: Winslow Press.

Chapter 3

Alzheimer's Society (2008) *Home From Home Report.* London: Alzheimer's Society.

Argyle, M. (1988) *Bodily Communications.* Madison, CT: International Universities Press.

Barnes, C. (2003) 'Chatter matters – advice on communication for carers.' *Journal of Dementia Care 11,* 5, 19–21.

Caris-Verhallen, W., Kerkstra, A. and Bensing, J. (1999) 'Factors related to nurse communication with elderly people.' *Journal of Advanced Nursing 30,* 5, 1106–1117.

Choices for Alzheimers (2009) *Alzheimers and Dementia Support.* Available at www. choicesforalzheimers.com/index.html, accessed on 13 December 2010.

Coaten, R. (2001) 'Exploring reminiscence through dance and movement.' *Journal of Dementia Care 9,* 5, 19–22.

Harley, T.A., Jessiman, L.J., MacAndrew, S.B. and Astell, A. (2008) 'I don't know what I know: Evidence of preserved semantic knowledge but impaired metalinguistic knowledge in adults with probable Alzheimer's disease.' *Aphasiology 22,* 3, 321–335.

Heathcote, J. (2009) *Memories are Made of This: Reminiscence Activities for Person-centred Care* (2nd edition). London: Alzheimer's Society.

Keene, J. (2000) 'Natural history of aggressive behaviour in dementia.' Alzheimer's Society newsletter, May. Summary of Keene, J., Hope, T., Fairburn, C., Jacoby, R., Gedling, K. and Ware, C. (1999) 'The natural history of aggressive behavior in dementia.' *International Journal of Geriatric Psychiatry 14,* 541–548.

Knocker, S. (2002) *Alzheimer's Society Book of Activities.* London: Alzheimer's Society.

Newson, P. (2010) 'Good communication at work can open the gateway to better relationships.' *Journal of Nursing and Residential Care 12,* 8, 366–369.

Sheard, D.M. (2009) *Nurturing our Emotions at Work in Dementia Care,* 'Feelings Matter Most' series, book 4. London: Alzheimer's Society.

Wilkins, A. and Mailoo, V.J. (2010) 'Care of the older person: a Hindu perspective.' *Journal of Nursing and Residential Care 12,* 5, 249–251.

WEB LINKS

CIRCA, Dementia Life (www.dementialife.com)

Pictures to Share (www.picturestoshare.co.uk)

Talking Mats (www.talkingmats.com)

SPECAL (www.specal.co.uk)

Chapter 4

Alzheimer's Society (2010) *This Is Me* leaflet. London: Alzheimer's Society. Available at http://alzheimers.org.uk/site/scripts/download_info. php?fileID=849, accessed on 13 December 2010.

Choices for Alzheimers (2009) *Alzheimers and Dementia Support.* Available at www. choicesforalzheimers.com/index.html, accessed on 13 December 2010.

Fisher, G., Arriaga, P., Less, C., Lee, J. and Ashpole, E. (2008) *The Residential Environment Impact Survey (REIS)* (version 2). Chicago, IL: Model of Human Occupation Clearinghouse, University of Illinois. Available at www.moho.uic.edu/REISinformation.html, accessed on 13 December 2010.

Folstein, M.F., Folstein, S.E. and McHugh, P.R. (1975) 'Mini-mental state: A practical method for grading the state of patients for the clinician.' *Journal of Psychiatric Research 12*, 189–198.

Heasman, D. and Salhortra, G. (2008) *UK Modified Interest Checklist*. Chicago, IL: Model of Human Occupation Clearinghouse, University of Illinois. Available at www.moho.uic.edu/mohorelatedrsrcs.html, accessed on 13 December 2010.

Hibberd, J.M. and Chia, S.H. (2007) 'Assessments – the contribution of occupational therapy.' *Journal of Nursing and Residential Care 9*, 6, 230–232.

Hodkinson, H.M. (1972) 'Evaluation of a mental test score for assessment of mental impairment in the elderly.' *Age and Ageing 1*, 4, 233–288.

Hopkins, H.L. and Smith, H.D. (eds) (1993) *Willard and Spackman's Occupational Therapy* (8th edition). Philadelphia, PA: JB Lippincott. Cited in A. Laver Fawcett (2007) *Principles of Assessment and Outcome Measurement for Occupational Therapists and Physiotherapists.* Hoboken, NJ: Wiley.

Laver Fawcett, A. (2007) *Principles of Assessment and Outcome Measurement for Occupational Therapists and Physiotherapists.* Hoboken, NJ: Wiley.

Law, M., Baptiste, S., Carswell, A., McColl, M.A., Polatajko, H. and Pollock, N. (2005) *Canadian Occupational Performance Measure* (4th edition). Toronto, Ontario: Canadian Association of Occupational Therapists.

Mayers, C. (2009) *The Mayers' Lifestyle Questionnaire (3)*. Available at www.mayersLSQ.org.uk, accessed on 13 December 2010.

National Mental Health Development Unit (NMHDU) (2010) *Mental Well-being Checklist*. London: NMHDU. Available at www.nmhdu.org.uk/silo/files/mental-wellbeing-checklist-a4.pdf, accessed on 13 December 2010.

Pool, J. (2008) *The Pool Activity Level (PAL) Instrument for Occupational Profiling: A Practical Resource for Carers of People with Cognitive Impairment* (3rd edition). London: Jessica Kingsley Publishers.

Prior, S. and Duncan, A.S. (2009) *Skills for Practice in Occupational Therapy.* Edinburgh: Churchill Livingstone.

Raphael, D., Renwick, R. and Brown, I. (1996) *Quality of Life Profile: Seniors Version (Full)*. Toronto, Ontario: Quality of Life Research Unit, University of Toronto. Available at www.utoronto.ca/qol/profile.htm, accessed on 13 December 2010.

School of Health Studies (2010) *Dementia Care Mapping*. Bradford: School of Health Studies, University of Bradford. Available at www.brad.ac.uk/health/dementia/DementiaCareMapping, accessed on 13 December 2010.

Whiting, S., Lincoln, N., Cockburn, J. and Bhavnani, G. (1985) *Rivermead Perceptual Assessment Battery III*. London: GL Assessment Limited.

Chapter 5

Creek, J. (2010) *The Core Concepts of Occupational Therapy*. London: Jessica Kingsley Publishers

Creek, J. and Bullock, A. (2008) 'Planning and Implementation.' In J. Creek and L. Lougher (eds) *Occupational Therapy and Mental Health*. Edinburgh: Elsevier Churchill Livingstone.

Hagedorn, R. (2000) *Tools for Practice in Occupational Therapy*. Edinburgh: Churchill Livingstone.

Hurtley, R. and Wenborn, J. (2000) *The Successful Activity Co-ordinator Training Pack*. London: Age Concern.

Luebben, A.J. and Royeen, C.B. (2010) 'An Acquisitional Frame of Reference.' In P. Kramer and J. Hinojosa (eds) *Frames of Reference for Pediatric Occupational Therapy*. Philadelphia, PA: Lippincott Williams and Wilkins.

Peck, C. and Hong, C.S. (1994) *Living Skills for Mentally Handicapped People*. London: Croom Helm.

Pool, J. (2008) *The Pool Activity Level (PAL) Instrument for Occupational Profiling: A Practical Resource for Carers of People with Cognitive Impairment* (3rd edition). London: Jessica Kingsley Publishers.

Chapter 6

Alzheimer's Society (2008) *Home From Home Report*. London: Alzheimer's Society.

Bender, M., Norris, A. and Bauckham, P. (1994) *Groupwork with the Elderly*. Bicester: Winslow Press.

Nordic Campbell Center (2008) 'Group activities help older people out of loneliness and isolation.' Copenhagen: SFi Campbell. Available at www.sfi.dk/Default.aspx?ID=454, accessed on 13 December 2010.

Robertson, L. and Fitzgerald, R. (2010) 'The conceptualisation of residential home environments: implications for occupational therapy.' *British Journal of Occupational Therapy 73*, 4, 170–177.

Toseland, R.W., Rivas, R.F. (2005) *An Introduction to Group Work Practice* (5th edition). Boston, MA: Ed Allyn and Bacon. Available at www.ablong.com, accessed on 13 December 2010.

Chapter 7

Bowden, A. and Lewthwaite, N. (2009) *The Activity Year Book.* London: Jessica Kingsley Publishers.

Cipriani, J., Haley, R., Moravec, E. and Young, H. (2010) 'Experience and meaning of group altruistic activities among long-term care residents.' *British Journal of Occupational Therapy 73*, 6, 269–276.

Halpern, A.R., Ly, J., Elkin-Frankston, S. and O'Connor, M.G. (2008) 'I know what I like: Stability of aesthetic preference in Alzheimer's patients.' *Brain and Cognition 66*, 1, 65–72.

Knocker, S. (2007) *Alzheimer's Society Book of Activities.* London: Alzheimer's Society.

MacGregor, K. and Driver, B. (2005) 'Activities that paint a thousand words.' *Journal of Dementia Care 13*, 6, 19–21.

McLean, V. (2004) 'Introducing crafts into the activity programme.' *Journal of Nursing and Residential Care 6*, 6, 284–285.

Mills, R. (2010) 'The beauty of recycling.' *Your Rubbish Your Choice*, summer, 15. Available at www.recyclefornorfolk.org.uk/content.asp?pid=200, accessed on 13 December 2010.

Truscott, M. (2004) 'Adapting leisure and creative activities for people with early stage dementia.' *Alzheimer's Quarterly 5*, 2, 92–102.

Wenborn, J. (2003a) 'The benefits of regular activity for care home residents.' *Journal of Nursing and Residential Care 5*, 3, 122–125.

Wenborn, J. (2003b) 'Encouraging creativity through arts and crafts.' *Journal of Nursing and Residential Care 5*, 8, 384–386.

Wenborn, J. (2004) 'Engaging people with dementia in care home activities.' *Journal of Nursing and Residential Care 6*, 3, 128–129.

Zoutewelle-Morris, S. (2010) 'Creative interaction with people in advanced dementia.' *Journal of Dementia Care 18*, 1, 20–22.

Chapter 8

Bittman, M.D., Berk, L.S., Felten, D.L., Westengard, J., Simonton, O.D., Pappas, J. and Ninehouser, M.D. (2001) 'Composite effects of group drumming music therapy on modulation of neuroendocrine-immune parameters in normal subjects.' *Alternatives Therapies 7*, 1, 38–47.

Chia, S.H., Heathcote, J., Quinn, P. and Plummer, M. (2005) 'Part three: Introduction to the Pabulum Wroxy Music group.' *Journal of Nursing and Residential Care 7*, 3, 125–127.

Cliff, S., Hancox, G., Staricoff, R. and Whitmore, C. (2008) *Singing and Health: A Systematic Mapping and Review of Non-clinical Research.* Canterbury: Sidney De Haan Research Centre for Arts and Health, Canterbury Christ Church University.

Hill, J. (2005) 'Music therapy for residents with neurological problems.' *Journal of Nursing and Residential Care 7*, 12, 563–564.

Jennings, S. (1986) *Creative Drama in Groupwork.* Bicester: Winslow Press.

Leary, S. (1994) *Activities for Personal Growth.* Sydney: Maclennan & Petty.

Munk-Madsen, N.M. (2001) 'Assessment in music therapy with clients suffering from dementia.' *Nordic Journal of Music Therapy 10*, 2, 205–208.

Pool, J. (2008) *The Pool Activity Level (PAL) Instrument for Occupational Profiling: A Practical Resource for Carers of People with Cognitive Impairment* (3rd edition). London: Jessica Kingsley Publishers.

Powell, H. and O Keefe, A. (2010) 'Weaving the threads together: Music therapy in care homes.' *Journal of Dementia Care 18*, 4, 24–28.

Roundabout (2007) *An Evaluation of Dramatherapy in a Care Home.* London: Roundabout.

Spelthorne Borough Council (2008) *Intergenerational Work in Spelthorne.* Spelthorne: Spelthorne Borough Council. Available at http://resources.cohesioninstitute.org.uk/GoodPractice/Projects/Project/Default.aspx?recordId=271, accessed on 20 February 2011.

Wenborn, J. (2003) 'The benefits of regular activity for care home residents.' *Journal of Nursing and Residential Care 5*, 3, 122–125.

Woods, M. (1982) *Music for Living.* Kidderminster: British Institute of Mental Handicap.

Web links

Alzheimer's Society (http://alzheimers.org.uk/)

Ladder to the Moon (www.ladder.to.themoon.co.uk

Lost Chord (www.lost-chord.org.uk)

Music for Life (www.wigmore-hall.org.uk/learning/in-the-community/music-for-life)

Chapter 9

Andrews, G.R. (2001) 'Promoting health and function in an ageing population.' *British Medical Journal 322*, 7288, 728–732.

Crichton, S. and Greenland, P. (1994) *First Moves – Movement Work with Very Young Children.* Leeds: Jabadao.

Heron, C. (1996) *The Relaxation Training Manual*. Bicester: Winslow Press.

Heymanson, C. (2009) 'Linking hands in circle dance.' *Journal of Dementia Care* *17*, 1, 13–14.

Manzoni, G.M., Pagnini, F., Castelnuovo, G. and Molinari, E. (2008) 'Relaxation training for anxiety: A ten-years systematic review with meta-analysis.' Available at www.biomedcentral.com/1471-244X/8/41, accessed on 17 February 2011.

Payne, H. (1997) *Creative Movement and Dance in GroupWork*. Bicester: Speechmark Publishing Ltd.

Yu, D.S.F., Lee, D.T.F., Woo, J. and Hui, E. (2007) 'Non-pharmacological interventions in older people with heart failure: Effects of exercise training and relaxation therapy.' *Gerontology 53*, 2, 74–81.

WEB LINKS

Active Norfolk (www.activenorfolk.org/fittogether)

Circle Dance (www.circledanceindementia.com)

EXTEND (www.extend.org.uk)

Green Candle Dance Company (www.greencandledance.com)

Jabadao (www.jabadao.org)

Medau Movement (www.medau.org.uk)

Vitalyz (www.vitalyz.co.uk)

Chapter 10

Chia, S.H. and Hibberd, J.M. (2009) 'Museum outreach: Making memory boxes.' *Journal of Dementia Care 17*, 1, 16–17.

Department of Health (2003) *Care Homes for Older People: National Minimum Standards*. London: The Stationery Office.

Department of Health (2009) *Living Well with Dementia: A National Strategy*. London: The Stationery Office.

Heathcote, J. (2009) *Memories are Made of This: Reminiscence Activities for Person-centred Care* (3rd edition). London: Alzheimer's Society.

Kitwood, T. (1997) *Dementia Reconsidered: The Person Comes First*. Buckingham: Open University Press.

School of Health Studies (2010) *Dementia Care Mapping*. Bradford: School of Health Studies, University of Bradford. Available at www.brad.ac.uk/ health/dementia/DementiaCareMapping, accessed on 13 September 2010.

Schweitzer, P. and Bruce, E. (2008) *Remembering Yesterday, Caring Today: Reminiscence in Dementia Care.* London: Jessica Kingsley Publishers.

Woods, B., Spector, A., Jones, C., Orrell, M. and Davies, S. (2005) 'Reminiscence therapy for dementia.' *Cochrane Database of Systematic Reviews,* April 18, 2, CD001120. Available at www.ncbi.nlm.nih.gov/pubmed/15846613, accessed on 13 December 2010.

WEB LINKS

Life Story Work (www.life-books.co.uk)

Chapter 11

Craig, C. and Mountain, G. (2007) *Lifestyle Matters: An Occupational Approach to Healthy Ageing.* Bicester: Speechmark Publishing Ltd.

Malouf, T. (2009) *The Hummingbird Bakery Cookbook.* London: Ryland, Peters & Small Ltd.

Mayers, C. (2009) *The Mayers' Lifestyle Questionnaire (3).* Available at www.mayersLSQ.org.uk, accessed on 13 December 2010.

Prosser, L. and Staiger, P. (2008) 'Older people's relationships with companion animals: A pilot study.' *Nursing Older People 20,* 3, 29–32.

Warr, P., Butcher, V. and Robertson, I. (2004) 'Activity and psychological well-being in older people.' *Ageing and Mental Health 8,* 2, 172–183.

Wells, D.L. (2007) 'Domestic dogs and human health: An overview.' *British Journal of Health Psychology 12,* 1, 145–156.

Chapter 12

Bender, M., Norris, A. and Bauckham, P. (1991) *Groupwork with the Elderly.* Bicester: Winslow Press.

Benham, L. (2007) 'What shall we do today?' *Journal of Dementia Care 15,* 4, 24–25.

Dynes, R. (1990) *Creative Games in Group Work.* Bicester: Winslow Press.

Hurtley, R. and Wenborn, J. (2000) *The Successful Activity Co-ordinator Training Pack.* London: Age Concern.

National Institute for Health and Clinical Excellence (NICE) (2006) *Dementia: Supporting People with Dementia and their Carers in Health and Social Care.* NICE Clinical Guideline 42. Available at www.nice.org.uk/guidance/cg42, accessed on 13 December 2010.

O'Donovan, S. (1996) *Simon's Nursing Assessment Manual.* Bicester: Winslow Press.

Pool, J. (2008) *The Pool Activity Level (PAL) Instrument for Occupational Profiling: A Practical Resource for Carers of People with Cognitive Impairment* (3rd edition). London: Jessica Kingsley Publishers.

Rimmer, L. (1982) *Reality Orientation – Principles and Practice.* Bicester: Winslow Press.

Spector, A., Thorgrimsen, L., Woods, B., Royan, S.D., Davies, S., Butterworth, M. and Orrell, M. (2003) 'Efficacy of an evidence-based cognitive stimulation therapy programme for people with dementia.' *British Journal of Psychiatry 183*, 3, 248–254.

Wenborn, J. (2003) 'Encouraging creativity through arts and crafts.' *Journal of Nursing and Residential Care 5*, 8, 384–388.

WEB LINKS

Age UK (www.ageuk.org.uk/IT)

CST – Cognitive stimulation therapy for dementia (www.cstdementia.com)

Learndirect (www.learndirect.co.uk)

Pass IT On (www.helppassiton.co.uk)

WebWise Basics (www.bbc.co.uk/webwise/courses)

Chapter 13

Chambers, M., Ryan, A. and Connors, S.L. (2001) 'Exploring the emotional support needs and coping strategies of family carers.' *Journal of Psychiatric and Mental Health Nursing 8*, 2, 99–106.

Charlesworth, G., Halford, J., Poland, F. and Vaughan, S. (2009) 'Carer Interventions in the Voluntary Sector.' In E. Moniz-Cook and J. Manthorpe (eds) *Early Psychosocial Interventions in Dementia: Evidence-Based Practice.* London: Jessica Kingsley Publishers.

Dröes, R.M., Meiland, F., De Lange, J., Vernooij-Dassen, M. and Van Tilburg, W. (2009) 'The Meeting Centres Support Programme.' In E. Moniz-Cook and J. Manthorpe (eds) *Early Psychosocial Interventions in Dementia: Evidence-Based Practice.* London: Jessica Kingsley Publishers.

Heathcote, J. and Chia, S.H. (2009) 'Groupwork as a tool to combat loneliness among older people: Initial observations.' *Groupwork 1*, 2, 121–130.

Heathcote, J., Newton, C. and Chia, S.H. (2007) 'A dementia service evaluated.' *Journal of Dementia Care 15*, 4, 13–14.

Mitchell, F. (1996) 'Carer support groups: The effects of organisational factors on the character of groups.' *Health and Social Care in the Community 4*, 2, 113–121.

Web links

Carers UK (www.carersuk.org)

Chapter 14

Bender, M., Norris, A. and Bauckham, P. (1991) *Groupwork With the Elderly.* Bicester: Winslow Press.

Cross, V. (1997) 'The professional development diary – A case study of one cohort of physiotherapy students.' *Physiotherapy 83*, 7, 375–383.

Laver Fawcett, A. (2007) *Principles of Assessment and Outcome Measurement for Occupational Therapists and Physiotherapists.* Hoboken, NJ: Wiley.

Law, M., Baptiste, S., Carswell, A., McColl, M.A., Polatajko, H. and Pollock, N. (2005) *Canadian Occupational Performance Measure* (4th edition). Toronto, Ontario: Canadian Association of Occupational Therapists.

NHS Institute for Innovation and Improvement (2008) *Quality and Service Improvement Tools: Plan, Do, Study, Act (PDSA).* Available at www.institute. nhs.uk/quality_and_service_improvement_tools/quality_and_service_ improvement_tools/plan_do_study_act.html, accessed on 13 December 2010.

Sheard, D.M. (2008) *Enabling Quality of Life: An Evaluation Tool,* 'Feelings Matter Most' series, book 2. London: Alzheimer's Society.

Stewart, S. (2004) 'The Place of Portfolios Within Continuing Professional Development.' In S.H. Chia and D. Harrison (eds) *Tools for Continuing Professional Development.* Trowbridge: Cromwell Press.

Subject Index

Author Index